AJPH

A PUBLICATION OF THE
AMERICAN PUBLIC HEALTH ASSOCIATION

AMERICAN JOURNAL of PUBLIC HEALTH
FEBRUARY 2024
Issue 2

THE LANGUAGES OF PUBLIC HEALTH

Words Matter, p. 140
Students' Perspectives, pp. 164–192
Cisgender Use, pp. 142 and 202

Also in this issue:

HISTORY
Vaccine Production & Skepticism, pp. 155 and 193

TELEHEALTH
Early Detection of COVID-19, pp. 146 and 218
Medication Abortion Care, pp. 152 and 241

TUBERCULOSIS
Among American Indians and Alaska Natives, pp. 149 and 226

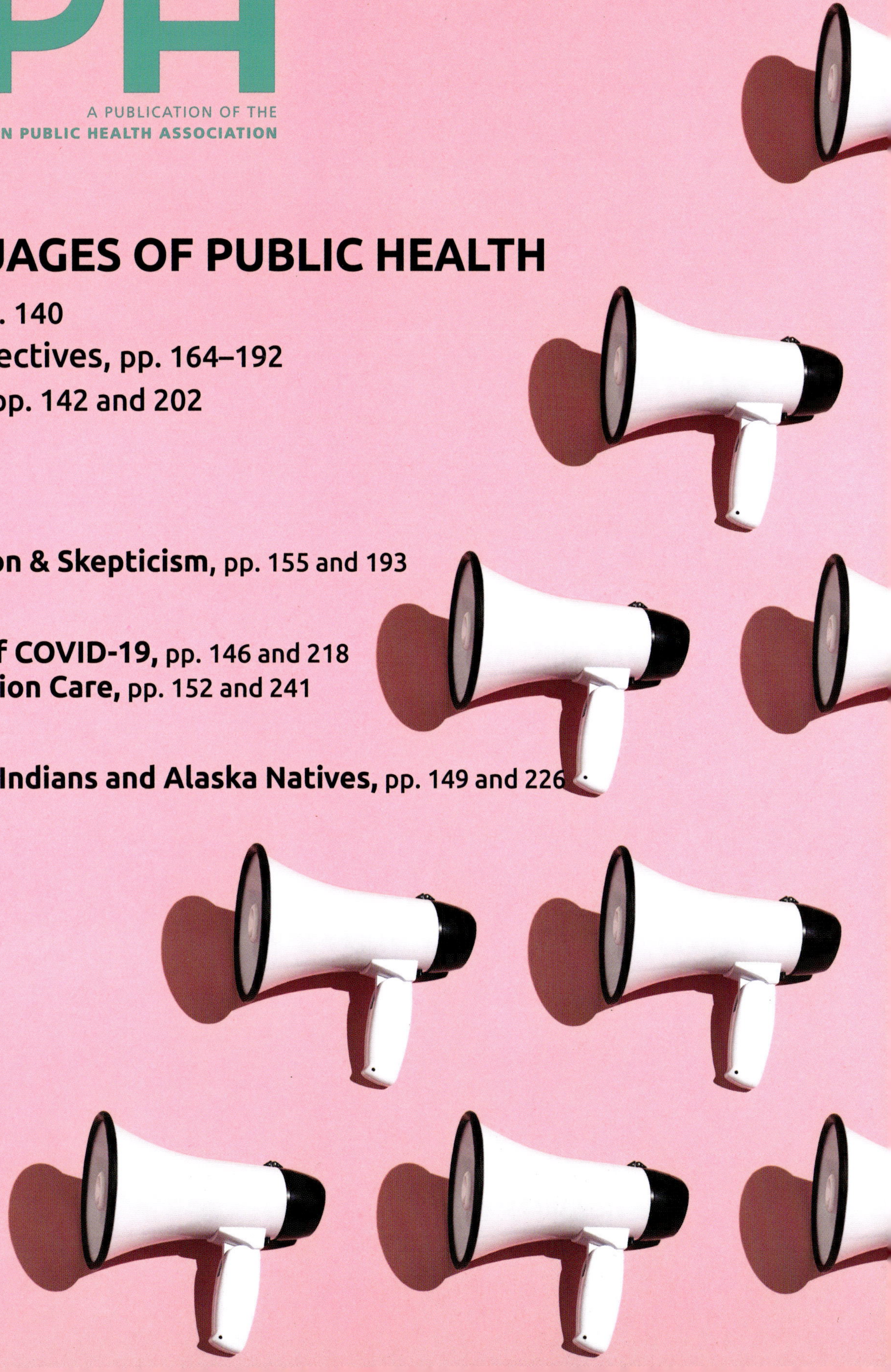

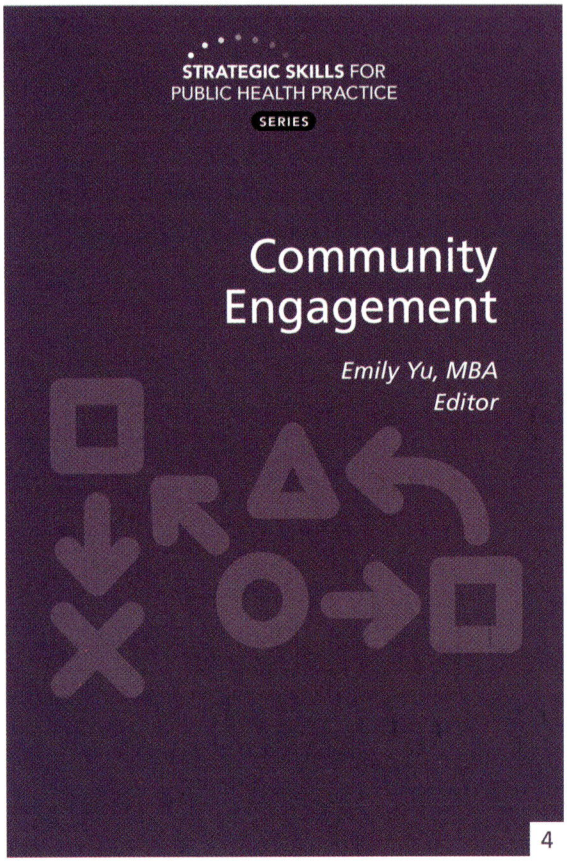

978-087553-3308, 108 PP, DIGITAL & SOFTCOVER

Community Engagement

Edited by Emily Yu, MBA

Community Engagement is the first book to be published from our new *Strategic Skills for Public Health Practice* series. This book brings the concept of community engagement to life through first-person stories, real-world examples and valuable insights from leaders across sectors. Curated specifically for public health practitioners and those interested in supporting community health, the book's chapters, guidance, and perspectives from the field will enhance readers' understanding of community-centered design and provide the tools to support organizational practices that drive better health for all.

APHABOOKSTORE.ORG

APHA PRESS

AN IMPRINT OF AMERICAN PUBLIC HEALTH ASSOCIATION

AMERICAN PUBLIC HEALTH ASSOCIATION
For science. For action. For health.

AJPH®, published monthly, is the official Journal of the American Public Health Association®, 800 I St NW, Washington, DC 20001-3710; (202) 777- APHA; TDD (202) 777-2500. APHA is a nongovernmental professional society founded in 1872, representing all disciplines and specialties in public health.

The *American Journal of Public Health*® (*AJPH*) (print ISSN: 0090-0036; electronic ISSN: 1541-0048), first published in 1911, is the official journal of the American Public Health Association® (APHA). The oldest and largest organization of public health professionals in the world, APHA represents approximately 30 000 members from more than 50 occupations of public health.

Submissions: Visit www.editorialmanager.com/ajph or ajph.edmgr.com for online manuscript preparation and submission guidelines. Contributions of original unpublished research, social science analyses, scholarly essays, critical commentaries, departments, and letters to the editor are welcome. Questions? Write ajph.submissions@apha.org or call APHA at (202) 777-2469.

Print plus online subscriptions: Institutional price (print copy with online access for a single institution and all authorized users, regardless of geographic location) varies by size of organization and ranges from $993–$1445 for US organizations, and $1073–$1526 for international organizations (air delivery); multiple campuses not permitted without special arrangement. Details of the tiered pricing system at https://subscriptionoffice.com/pages/apha-landing-page. To order, write apha.subscriptions@apha.org.

Online-only subscriptions: Institutional price for one institution and its authorized users (regardless of geographic location) is $878–$1307. To order, write apha.subscriptions@apha.org. For academic consortia or multisite corporate subscriptions, contact apha.subscriptions@apha.org.

Print-only subscriptions: Institutional price is US $701, $782 international.

Back print issues: A limited number of print issues are for sale. Single copies are US $49, $55 international (air delivery). Shipping included; prepay only. To order, write apha.subscriptions@apha.org.

Reprints: For prices and ordering information on 50 or more reprints, check the Reprints section at www.ajph.org. To order smaller quantities of reprints (rush delivery), use the "Purchase Article" link on the article site itself.

Electronic access: Online articles more than 10 years old are available free for personal use at www.ajph.org. Recent articles are available through pay-per-view: single PDF article for $24, single issue access for 24 hours for $33, or entire site access for 24 hours for $38.

Postal information: Periodicals postage paid at Washington, DC, and additional mailing offices. Postmaster: Send address changes to American Journal of Public Health, 800 I St NW, Washington, DC 20001-3710.

Address changes: Send to AJPH, Membership Department (members) or AJPH Subscriptions (subscribers), APHA, 800 I St NW, Washington, DC 20001-3710. Or write to membership.mail@apha. org (members) or apha.subscriptions@apha.org (subscribers).

Indexes: Publications that index or abstract articles from AJPH include the following: Ageline, Assia (Applied Social Science Index and Abstracts), Biological Abstracts, Chemical Abstracts, CINAHL, Criminal Justice Abstracts, EMBASE, EMCare, Environmental Abstracts, e-psyche, ERIC, ETOH (Alcohol and Alcohol Problems Science Database), Excerpta Medica, Food Science and Technology, General Science Index, Grateful Med, Hospital Literature Index, Human Resources Abstracts, International Pharmaceutical Abstracts (IPA), Medline, Physical Education Index, Pollution Abstracts, Psychological Abstracts, PsychINFO, Safety Science Abstracts, Sage Family Studies Abstracts, Sage Human Resources Abstracts, Science Citation Index, SCOPUS, SIIC Data Bases, Social Work Research and Abstracts, and Statistical Reference Index (SRI)/LexisNexis.

AJPH
A PUBLICATION OF THE
AMERICAN PUBLIC HEALTH ASSOCIATION

COVER: To (re)build trust and advance health for all, we must become fluent in "The Languages of Public Health." This cover image captures the essence of the special section, highlighting that the power of public health lies not just in words but also in the method we choose to share our messages. We hope this special section promotes the fluency of deliberative language, mindful framing, and inclusive communication strategies needed to find common ground and advance equitable health.

Cover concept and image selection by Aleisha Kropf. Image by DeBenitostock/Getty printed with permission.

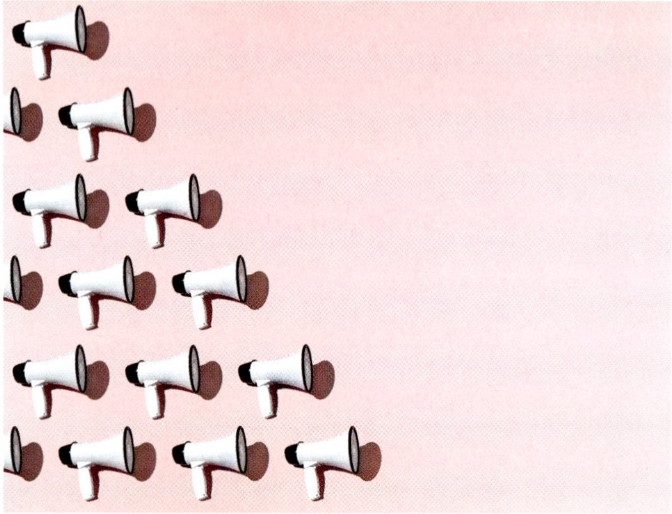

APHA
AMERICAN PUBLIC HEALTH ASSOCIATION
For science. For action. For health.

Promoting public health research, policy, practice, and education is the *AJPH* mission. As we widen our scope to embrace global issues, we also sharpen our focus to support the needs of public health practitioners. We invite contributions of original unpublished research, opinion and commentary, and letters to the editor.

The *Journal* is printed on acid-free recycled paper.

AJPH February 2024, Vol. 114, No. 2

OPEN ACCESS · ONLINE ONLY · PODCAST · DATA SUPPLEMENT AVAILABLE

EDITOR'S CHOICE

140 Words Matter: The Languages of Public Health
B. E. Williams, T. J. Fuller, P. Juturu, F. N. Rashoka, J. Vasquez, and D. Oluwemimo; AJPH Student Think Tank

OPINIONS, IDEAS, & PRACTICE

EDITORIALS

142 Cisgender Privilege in Public Health Research
A. S. Keuroghlian

144 Thinking Broadly About Public Health Data
J. Levi

146 Harnessing Telehealth: Improving Epidemic Prediction and Response
G. Chowell and A. Lawson

149 Tuberculosis in US Indigenous Communities: A Need for Public Health Prioritization
L. Cilloni and D. W. Dowdy

152 Opportunities for Increasing Access to Person-Centered Abortion Care Through Telehealth
E. Munson and K. S. Hall

155 Vaccine Hesitancy, Pharmaceutical Marketing, and Mistrusted Messengers
J. Colgrove

158 Adolescent Mental Health and Well-Being: A Public Health of Consequence, February 2024
F. Kapadia

PERSPECTIVES

161 The Public Health Crisis State of Transgender Health Care and Policy
A. J. Restar, E. K. Layland, B. Davis, H. Thompson, and C. Streed Jr

THE LANGUAGES OF PUBLIC HEALTH

164 The Languages of Public Health: Student Perspectives on Terms, Communities, and Language
F. N. Rashoka, J. Vasquez, B. E. Williams, T. J. Fuller, P. Juturu, and D. Oluwemimo

166 The Languages of Public Health: Avoiding a Modern-Day "Tower of Babel"
R. J. Kim-Farley

168 The Power of Poetry: Rethinking How We Use Language in Global Health Research
L. L. Woodson

170 "We're Here, We're Queer, Get Used to It": Advancing LGBTQ+-Inclusive Language in Public Health
T. D. Harvey

173 The Resignation on Race
C. A. Carter

175 Public Health's Language Incompatibility With Veterans
T. Henson

177 Vulnerabilized: Revisiting the Language of the Vulnerable Populations Framework
C. M. Garrett and R. Altman

180 Public Health Preparedness Practitioners: Fluent in Disaster
C. Kuddes

183 Medical Etymology: A Journey of Identity
C. Mitchell

184 One Afternoon at a Vaccination Clinic
F. E. Muller

186 When Public Health Terms Become Vernacular
N. J. Matangi

188 Imagery as a Participatory Tool of Resilience for Marginalized Persons
G. I. A. Adan

190 Unseen and Unheard: Increasing the Visibility of Limited English Proficiency Individuals Through a Language Justice Framework
T. Jilu

RESEARCH & ANALYSIS

HISTORY

193 From Farms to Pharma: A "Natural" History of Vaccine Production and Vaccine Skepticism
T. Lanzarotta

PERSPECTIVES FROM THE SOCIAL SCIENCES

202 Common Patterns of Cisgender Use in Public Health Articles and Their Implications for Gender Inclusivity Efforts, 2013–2020
A. Esacove

SURVEILLANCE

209 Regulations and Funding to Create Enterprise Architecture for a Nationwide Health Data Ecosystem
G. Seidman, A. AlKasir, K. Ricker, J. T. Lane, A. B. Zink, and M. A. Williams

218 Use of Telehealth Information for Early Detection: Insights From the COVID-19 Pandemic
S. Haenchen, B. McCabe, W. J. Mack, J. N. Doctor, J. A. Linder, S. D. Persell, J. Tibbels, and D. Meeker

OPEN-THEMED RESEARCH

226 Racial and Ethnic Disaggregation of Tuberculosis Incidence and Risk Factors Among American Indian and Alaska Native Persons—United States, 2001–2020
Y. P. Springer, T. D. Filardo, R. S. Woodruff, and J. L. Self

237 COVID-19 Vaccination Rates Among North Dakota Residents Who Gave Birth Between April 1, 2021, and July 15, 2022
O. Aguilar and M. Woinarowicz

241 Patient Acceptability of Telehealth Medication Abortion Care in the United States, 2021–2022: A Cohort Study
L. R. Koenig, J. Ko, E. S. Valladares, F. M. Coeytaux, E. Wells, C. R. Lyles, and U. D. Upadhyay

BACKMATTER

LETTERS & RESPONSES

251 Unpacked Cochrane Review on Masks: A Further Look
J. M. Kivelä

252 Gurbaxani et al. Respond
B. M. Gurbaxani, A. N. Hill, and P. Patel

OTHER DEPARTMENTS

256 Subscription Form

Words Matter: The Languages of Public Health

See also The Languages of Public Health, pp. 164–192.

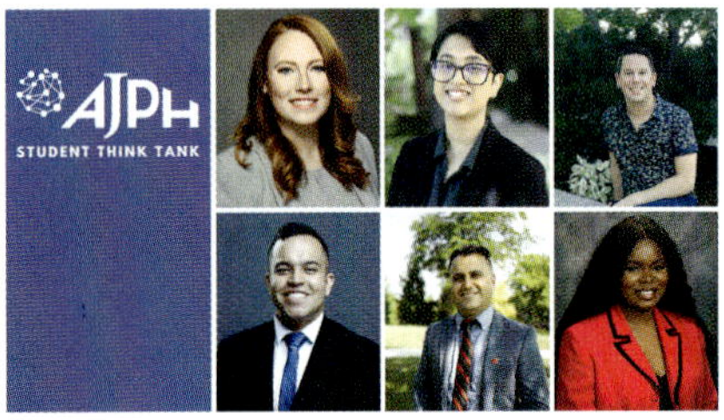

Blair E. Williams, MPA, MBA, CPH, Tyler J. Fuller, MTS, MPH, CHES, Preeti Juturu, Falah Nayif Rashoka, RN, MS, CPH, MPH, Jesus Vasquez, MS, MPH, and Damilola Oluwemimo; *AJPH* Student Think Tank

The languages of public health are complex and often politicized, making it difficult for public health practitioners to craft effective health messaging, build trust, and navigate funding opportunities. In the current climate—characterized by partisan politics, misinformation, skepticism, and heightened disparities, all intensified by the COVID-19 crisis—these tasks are particularly daunting. Moreover, the integration of artificial intelligence (AI) has precipitated changes in the public health vocabulary with growing concerns of algorithmic bias and data quality limitations. Given the potential to be either unifying or polarizing, the languages of public health matter as we seek to (re)build trust and advance public health.

Language shapes our world, how we speak, and how we think. Language often works unconsciously in the background of our minds, and it is a lens through which we see, interpret, and act in the world. As such, it also shapes health-seeking behaviors and policy (http://bit.ly/46cK42G). Differences in social position (e.g., being privileged or marginalized), as well as political lean, also shape language and worldviews across physical, social, and even digital spaces. Different understandings of technical terms can also lead to alarm and distrust, such as when the general US public interpreted epidemiological "surveillance" as a loss of privacy (https://bit.ly/46ed5Lj). Epidemiologists use this word in a specific way that is different from the colloquial meaning. Even if both epidemiologists and the general public are speaking in a common language (e.g., English), one's background knowledge and life experiences are fundamental to making different associations and interpretations. In many ways, it may feel like another language altogether.

The language of public health consists of evolving terms to describe theoretical constructs, populations, organizations, therapies, and diseases. These terms are often driven by science, culture, geography, politics, history, and technology. We routinely use terms in our field that might seem intuitive yet miss the step of translating technical jargon into plain language. For example, at the peak of the COVID-19 pandemic, technical terms like "herd

Continued on page 141...

HISTORY CORNER

10 YEARS AGO

Ethical Issues in Conducting Research With Deaf Populations

[C]ultural naïvetë and lack of language fluency create a host of barriers and ethical dilemmas for many health researchers who work with minority, underserved, and vulnerable populations. Collaborating with underrepresented communities requires researchers to demonstrate creativity, mutual respect, flexibility, compassion, cultural competency, and patience in their work. . . . Few health researchers understand the cultural values held by the Deaf community or even know ASL [American Sign Language]. The lack of linguistic and cultural concordance places the population at high risk for poor research engagement and inaccessible informed-consent processes and research materials. This perpetuates a long-standing history of fear, mistrust, and frustration of deaf ASL users with biomedical researchers and their research studies.

From *AJPH*, December 2013, p. 2174

13 YEARS AGO

Community-Based Participatory Research to Improve Health Equity

[T]he third challenge [for translational research] is language, which includes incompatible discourse between the academy and the community, and the power of naming, immunity" and "comorbidity" rapidly entered the public vernacular; however, the average person may not interpret these terms as they were intended in the field. Additionally, the term "herd" might be lost in translation, whereby the literal interpretation might lead people to think they were being compared with animals. On the other hand, a misguided attempt to oversimplify a nuanced topic may lead the audience to misinterpret the key message or inadvertently mischaracterize a subpopulation with potentially stigmatizing narratives. This lack of clear communication can result in a wide array of problems, from poor adherence to public health guidelines to the spread of misinformation. Furthermore, ineffective public health messaging intensifies stress, stigma, and cognitive bias, whereas a well-crafted public health message considers the audience while framing issues for action (https://bit.ly/47cajrc).

Accessible and inclusive language is required when considering the diverse health needs of populations and communities. Alarming disparities and trends associated with chronic conditions, mortality, and life expectancy all signal a need for equitable access to patient-centered care. Black, Indigenous, and People of Color; members of the lesbian, gay, bisexual, transgender, and questioning community; and people with disabilities are impacted by persistent systemic inequities and injustices that contribute to feelings of mistrust in health care systems. For those addressing health inequities and trust deficits, the delivery of socially and culturally appropriate care is strengthened with inclusive language and steps to mitigate health literacy or language barriers.

For those assessing and addressing disparities at the population level, data equity practices using equitable language reduce the risk of contributing to harmful narratives or perpetuating disinformation around health disparities. However, in scenarios where discourse exists because of political climate, it can be daunting to harmoniously navigate phrases that are agreeable with both politics and best practices. The navigation of evolving, polarizing, stigmatizing, or confusing terms is an ongoing exercise for those working to (re)build trust and advance health. However, the use of deliberative language in public health (https://bit.ly/49wT45n) and evolution of natural language processing in artificial intelligence (https://bit.ly/3MHLISY) are examples of how language can be leveraged in the pursuit of more equitable and healthier nation.

A cyclical relationship exists between bias and public health languages, and this is well demonstrated in policy. Often the use of culturally appropriate terms is considered "politically correct;" ironically, the terms favored in policy may not actually be the best choice of words to describe a concept or population. In late 2017, the US Centers for Disease Control and Prevention received instruction not to use seven words in its 2019 budget appropriation request: diversity, transgender, vulnerable, fetus, entitlement, evidence-based, and science-based (https://bit.ly/3QWVjHQ). After this request, many public health officials resisted this perceived attempt at censorship and effort to dehumanize marginalized populations. The potential exclusion of these seven words in the budget appropriation might have had serious funding and ethical implications.

The interconnected nature of public health and language has implications in our collective effort to advance health in the United States and on an international scale. Our research and practice are strengthened by our ability to effectively communicate and connect with our audience. By placing importance on the languages of public health, we are well-positioned to (re)build trust and serve the very public we aim to protect. AJPH

DOI: https://doi.org/10.2105/AJPH.2023.307540

HISTORY CORNER

which encompasses such commonly used terms as "institutionalization" or "collaborators." These terms can unwittingly trigger resistance and historical memories of assimilationist policies or betrayal. . . . The use of language is closely tied to knowledge dominance, with [community-based participatory research] advocating changes in research discourse—that is, from "research subject" to "research participant," or from "targeting community members" to "engaging community partners." Ongoing dialogue with partners about discourse specific to local values remains critical; for example, the language of "institutionalizing" programs can bring up historical trauma from government, schools, or academic institutions that have caused damage in communities of color.

From *AJPH*, Supplement 1, 2010, p. S40

Cisgender Privilege in Public Health Research

Alex S. Keuroghlian, MD, MPH

ABOUT THE AUTHOR

The author is with Harvard Medical School, Boston, MA; The Fenway Institute, Fenway Health, Boston; and the Department of Psychiatry, Massachusetts General Hospital, Boston.

See also Esacove, p. 202.

Society grants privilege automatically, in the form of rights or advantages, to members of certain dominant groups and not to others.[1] Examining such privilege can be uncomfortable for those who hold it. Privilege does not necessarily mean that people have lived an easy life or that they have an intention to deprive or harm others. Within an intersectionality framework, many of us hold privilege in certain ways and oppressed or minoritized identities in other ways, for example based on our race, ethnicity, language, religion, age, sexual orientation, economic status, ability, or citizenship.[2]

As Anne Esacove points out in the new article "Common Patterns of Cisgender Use in Public Health Articles and Their Implications for Gender Inclusivity Efforts, 2013–2020" (p. 202), the term cisgender has historically been a marker of normative gender and of systems of social power built on the false assumption that gender identity will always align with societal expectations according to the sex assigned at birth. Indeed, the Latin prefix cis means on the same side, in this case indicating that gender identity and sex assigned at birth align on the basis of societal expectations. In contrast, the term transgender includes the Latin prefix trans, which means opposite side, indicating that, according to societal expectations, gender identity and sex assigned at birth do not align.

In recent years, the adjective cisgender has referred increasingly to individuals whose gender identities align with traditional expectations based on their sex assigned at birth. As Esacove demonstrates, great variability exists in public health research regarding the context, methodology, and application of cisgender demographic data collection and utilization.

Esacove's article offers opportunities for improvement in public health data collection with regard to cisgender considerations, including explicitness and clarity around objectives, theoretical frameworks, definitions, and protocols for participant gender identity determination; consistent use of the term cisgender throughout all sections of individual publications, on par with use of transgender, and across studies on health outcomes beyond those focused on gender and sexually diverse people or related health topics; innovation of best practices for research participants to self-identify as cisgender with the option to select all gender identity response options that may apply; and study of gendered sociopolitical structures that influence health through cissexist effects on people of all gender identities and expressions. In addition, gender itself is multidimensional and certain dimensions of gender, which we must continue to delineate empirically, may be more relevant for some public health studies than for others.

Although we might hypothesize that people who hold cisgender privilege would be reluctant to acknowledge this as public health research participants, there is cause for optimism based on existing studies. Since 2016, the Health Resources and Services Administration Bureau of Primary Health Care has required reporting of patient gender identity data by all US federally qualified health centers (FQHCs).[3] From 2016 to 2021, completeness of patient gender identity data reporting by FQHCs more than doubled, from 37.2% to 76%, with most respondents not identifying as transgender or gender diverse.[4] More complete and accurate patient gender identity documentation has in turn enabled researchers to begin harnessing electronic health record data sets at FQHCs for the study of pressing public health concerns.[5]

Completeness of patient gender identity data reporting is higher in localities with less structural stigma, specifically in US municipalities with stronger gender identity nondiscrimination laws.[6] Thus, protective governmental policies pertaining to gender identity are likely to foster favorable environments for gender identity disclosure and data collection in public health research. Implementation of patient-centered and trauma-informed care across health care organizations and systems may also decrease stigma and thereby further promote completeness of gender identity disclosure within public health research. If public health studies afford research participants the chance to answer well-explained gender identity questions in psychologically safe environments that minimize

AJPH February 2024, Vol. 114, No. 2

stigma, this may even prompt some participants to contemplate, for the first time, whether they are indeed as cisgender as they may have once assumed.

Future refinements in measurement of cisgender phenomena relevant to public health can build on, and integrate with, current health care guidelines and recommended practices. Detailed protocols exist for planning and implementing gender identity data collection within electronic health records, which requires careful, multifaceted change management that engages all relevant stakeholders.[7] When considering experiences across the life span, developmentally appropriate tailoring of patient gender identity questions can occur for children, adolescents, and adults.[8]

Moreover, although often discussed in the context of transgender and gender diverse people, gender-affirming care is in fact necessary for patients of all gender identities, including cisgender patients. Electronic health records can support high-quality gender-affirming care through anatomical inventories, clinical decision support tools, and features that facilitate population health management to ensure measurement-based continuous quality improvement.[9] The National Committee for Quality Assurance, the developer of the Healthcare Effectiveness Data and Information Set, which most American health insurance plans utilize, is now integrating gender-based quality measurement.[10] This will mark a paradigm shift that is poised to advance health equity.

For public health research to do the same, development of gender-related measures, design of studies, interpretation of findings, and reporting of conclusions must occur with meaningful involvement of transgender and gender diverse community members, who are most harmed by entrenched cisgender systems of power.[11] For example, some public health experts have been skeptical of nonprobability sampling methods, which utilize nonrandom research participant selection, owing to questions about whether these approaches can yield generalizable and externally valid results. Nonprobability sampling, however, facilitates recruiting larger transgender and gender diverse participant sample sizes with sufficient power to conduct important subgroup analyses and answer specific public health questions of high priority for transgender and gender diverse communities.[12]

In the years ahead, public health research must keep up with, and be responsive to, rapidly evolving concepts and terminology related to gender and sex. Public health professionals have the choice to approach this linguistic, sociocultural, and health care revolution with apprehension, frustration, and resistance or instead with openness, curiosity, and innovation. The former is a reaction rooted in privilege. The latter is a path to more inclusive public health for all. AJPH

CORRESPONDENCE

Correspondence should be sent to Alex S. Keuroghlian, MD, MPH, The Fenway Institute, Fenway Health, Boston, MA 02115 (e-mail: akeuroghlian@mgb.org). Reprints can be ordered at http://www.ajph.org by clicking the "Reprints" link.

PUBLICATION INFORMATION

Full Citation: Keuroghlian AS. Cisgender privilege in public health research. *Am J Public Health*. 2024;114(2):142–143.

Acceptance Date: November 20, 2023

DOI: https://doi.org/10.2105/AJPH.2023.307542

CONFLICTS OF INTEREST

The author declares royalties from McGraw Hill as editor of a textbook on transgender and gender diverse health care and royalties from the American Psychiatric Association as editor of a textbook on gender-affirming psychiatric care.

REFERENCES

1. *Merriam-Webster Dictionary*. Privilege (noun). Available at: https://www.merriam-webster.com/dictionary/privilege. Accessed January 3, 2024.
2. Bowleg L. Evolving intersectionality within public health: from analysis to action. *Am J Public Health*. 2021;111(1):88–90. https://doi.org/10.2105/AJPH.2020.306031
3. Grasso C, Goldhammer H, Funk D, et al. Required sexual orientation and gender identity reporting by US health centers: first-year data. *Am J Public Health*. 2019;109(8):1111–1118. https://doi.org/10.2105/AJPH.2019.305130
4. Liu M, King D, Mayer KH, Grasso C, Keuroghlian AS. Sexual orientation and gender identity data completeness at US federally qualified health centers, 2020 and 2021. *Am J Public Health*. 2023;113(8):883–892. https://doi.org/10.2105/AJPH.2023.307323
5. McDowell MJ, King DS, Gitin S, et al. Alcohol use disorder treatment in sexually and gender diverse patients: a retrospective cohort study. *J Clin Psychiatry*. 2023;84(5):23m14812. https://doi.org/10.4088/JCP.23m14812.
6. Almazan AN, King D, Grasso C, et al. Sexual orientation and gender identity data collection at US health centers: impact of city-level structural stigma in 2018. *Am J Public Health*. 2021;111(11):2059–2063. https://doi.org/10.2105/AJPH.2021.306414
7. Grasso C, McDowell MJ, Goldhammer H, Keuroghlian AS. Planning and implementing sexual orientation and gender identity data collection in electronic health records. *J Am Med Inform Assoc*. 2019;26(1):66–70. https://doi.org/10.1093/jamia/ocy137
8. Goldhammer H, Grasso C, Katz-Wise SL, Thomson K, Gordon AR, Keuroghlian AS. Pediatric sexual orientation and gender identity data collection in the electronic health record. *J Am Med Inform Assoc*. 2022;29(7):1303–1309. https://doi.org/10.1093/jamia/ocac048
9. Grasso C, Goldhammer H, Thompson J, et al. Optimizing gender-affirming medical care through anatomical inventories, clinical decision support, and population health management in electronic health record systems. *J Am Med Inform Assoc*. 2021;28(11):2531–2535. https://doi.org/10.1093/jamia/ocab080
10. National Committee for Quality Assurance. NCQA updates and releases new quality measures for HEDIS 2023 with a focus on health equity. Available at: https://www.ncqa.org/news/ncqa-updates-releases-new-quality-measures-for-hedis-2023-with-a-focus-on-health-equity-stratifying-measures-by-race-ethnicity-and-affirming-gender-identity-helps-tackle-health-disparities. Accessed October 5, 2023.
11. Keuroghlian AS, Keatley J, Shaikh S, Radix AE. The context, science and practice of gender-affirming care. *Nat Med*. 2022;28(12):2464–2467. https://doi.org/10.1038/s41591-022-02082-w
12. Turban JL, Almazan AN, Reisner SL, et al. The importance of non-probability samples in minority health research: lessons learned from studies of transgender and gender diverse mental health. *Transgend Health*. 2023;8(4):302–306. https://doi.org/10.1089/trgh.2021.0132

Thinking Broadly About Public Health Data

Jeffrey Levi, PhD

ABOUT THE AUTHOR

Jeffrey Levi is professor emeritus of health policy and management, Milken Institute School of Public Health, George Washington University, Washington, DC.

See also Seidman et al., p. 209.

As we think about building a national public health data infrastructure, we must keep in mind three critical issues: (1) our definition of public health data must be driven by the goal of advancing equity and thus must include the multiple factors that affect individual and population health, including social factors that are rarely part of traditional health and disease surveillance; (2) a data system must be built in a modernized public health system focused on foundational public health capabilities, embracing a workforce that can analyze data and mobilize government agencies and communities to address the implications of the data; and (3) our design and our use of public health data must be driven by and accessible to communities and the multisector partnerships that are the centerpiece of improving population and community health.

In this issue of *AJPH*, Seidman et al. (p. 209) lay an excellent groundwork in their description of the need for a national health data ecosystem. Their description of a national rather than a federal data system accurately reflects both the constitutional and the political reality of public health in the United States. This is consistent with the work of the Commonwealth Fund Commission on a National Public Health System, which I helped staff.[1] The Commission said that we can build from the current state, tribal, local, and territorial (STLT) public health structure by embracing foundational public health capabilities as a minimum standard for all STLTs—agreeing with the authors that this can be driven by federal leadership and incentivized with federal funding but also arguing that in exchange for this federal investment, there must be strong accountability that ensures that every US resident is served by these foundational public health capabilities. (Assessment and surveillance is one of the foundational capabilities.) The Commission argued that this can be done with a series of measures, including using a modernized accreditation system that is tied to increased federal funding. Whether it is a data system or other foundational capabilities, model regulations and incentivized funding are necessary but insufficient.[2]

BROADENING PUBLIC HEALTH DATA

As Seidman et al. remind us, our understanding of what drives health outcomes increasingly reflects social determinants of health. Indeed, to have a clear understanding of the health of a community or a population, we must look at traditional public health data, health care data, and social needs. Too many discussions about modernizing public health data systems focus on the relationship between public health and health care and their interoperability. This is critical, without a doubt, and in itself raises very complex policy and regulatory questions. But increasingly, our public health work is driven by a variety of equity indexes that also attempt to measure health-related social needs (e.g., housing and food insecurity) although we have not taken on the policy and funding issues associated with collecting social needs data. The work of the Data Across Systems for Health project is one example of an effort to develop such a cross-sector model.[3]

Given this, we must move beyond collecting data about social needs to also document access to social services that address those social needs—just as we document access to health care services, not just what illnesses are prevalent in a community. This is one of the biggest gaps in our current ability to understand inequities in the United States and will require building the data capacity (and associated funding and privacy policies) of a large network of social services agencies to participate in a more robust public health data ecosystem.

SUPPORTING DATA COLLECTION AND EFFECTIVE USE

Ethically, public health data collection should be premised on the assumption that we will act on what the data tell us to improve individual and community health. But for this to happen, public health needs a workforce that can analyze and translate the data into meaningful policy and programs, which requires an investment in technology. The workforce must also be able to perform surveillance and epidemiology and have the many necessary foundational public health capabilities, including the

AJPH February 2024, Vol. 114, No. 2

ability to deliver the broad array of foundational public health programs.

The Commission recommended two levels of investment in this regard: $4.5 billion in annual federal funding to give the STLTs the resources needed to close the current gap in their ability to deliver on the foundational public health capabilities[4] and $36.7 billion over 10 years specifically for building a modernized public health data system, a cost estimated by the Healthcare Information Management Systems Society.[5]

Why such a high level of investment? The Public Health National Center for Innovation performed a comprehensive assessment of the current US workforce and estimated that there is a shortfall of 80 000 full-time employees needed to meet basic community public health functions across the STLTs. Of that number, 9000 full-time employees would be needed for the assessment (surveillance, epidemiology, etc.) function alone.[6]

In a decentralized public health system, one could ask why this funding should be principally a federal responsibility. Without the federal government funding and setting expectations with regard to minimum capacity of the STLTs across the country, we would reinforce inequities because of varied capacity to address everyday problems, and we would have differential ability to respond to epidemics and other national threats that cannot be contained within borders of jurisdictions less willing or able to build comprehensive public health capacity.

DESIGN AND USE OF PUBLIC HEALTH DATA

One of the foundational public health capabilities is community partnerships. This reflects a long-standing understanding in public health but is even more central as we increase our focus on equity and social determinants of health. We have come to understand that granular data—those at the zip code and census tract levels—are critical to understanding the nonmedical drivers of health and identifying inequities that aggregated data might mask. What data are collected and how the data are translated into action at the community level must be driven by community voice and the multisector partners that must come together to solve the problems at the local level.

The Robert Wood Johnson Foundation's National Commission to Transform Public Health Data Systems provides a detailed model for engaging communities in designing public health data system.[7] Although this may seem aspirational, especially given the current state of our data infrastructure, across the country public health agencies and philanthropy are engaging in supporting creative partnerships—often called "accountable communities for health"—that can be the springboard for cross-sector responses that can build strong, resilient communities that reduce inequities.[8,9]

CONCLUSIONS

Public health is at a crossroads. In the postpandemic environment, there is an understanding that our public health system is in desperate need of change while public health also faces diminished public trust. An approach to public health modernization, including data modernization, that builds capacity while engaging community may well be the formula that creates the political will to sustain a national public health (and data) ecosystem. AJPH

CORRESPONDENCE

Correspondence should be sent to Jeffrey Levi, PhD, Department of Health Policy and Management, 2175 K St NW, 5th floor, Washington, DC 20052 (e-mail: jlevi@gwu.edu). Reprints can be ordered at http://www.ajph.org by clicking the "Reprints" link.

PUBLICATION INFORMATION

Full Citation: Levi J. Thinking broadly about public health data. *Am J Public Health*. 2024;114(2): 144–145.

Acceptance Date: November 22, 2023.

DOI: https://doi.org/10.2105/AJPH.2023.307548

CONFLICTS OF INTEREST

The author has no conflicts of interest to declare.

REFERENCES

1. Commonwealth Fund. Meeting America's public health challenge. June 21, 2022. Available at: https://www.commonwealthfund.org/publications/fund-reports/2022/jun/meeting-americas-public-health-challenge. Accessed October 19, 2023.
2. Public Health Accreditation Board Center for Innovation. The foundational public health services. 2023. Available at: https://phaboard.org/center-for-innovation/public-health-frameworks/the-foundational-public-health-services. Accessed October 19, 2023.
3. Data Across Sectors for Health. The state of the field of multisector data sharing for community health: report of the all in national inventory 2.0. 2023. Available at: https://static1.squarespace.com/static/6320ea657f0aff58aef9a3ca/t/6512e97f05b3150401fe8837/1695738240333/DASH_National_Inventory_Report_2.pdf. Accessed October 19, 2023.
4. DeSalvo K, Parekh A, Hoagland GW, et al. Developing a financing system to support public health infrastructure. *Am J Public Health*. 2019;109(10):1358–1361. [Erratum in: *Am J Public Health*. 2020;110(9):e15]. https://doi.org/10.2105/AJPH.2019.305214
5. Healthcare Information Management Systems Society. Public health information and technology infrastructure: modernization funding report. April 29, 2022. Available at: https://www.himss.org/resources/public-health-information-and-technology-infrastructure-modernization-funding-report. Accessed October 19, 2023.
6. de Beaumont Foundation. Staffing up: workforce levels needed to provide basic public health services for all Americans. October 2021. Available at: https://debeaumont.org/wp-content/uploads/2021/10/Staffing-Up-FINAL.pdf. Accessed October 19, 2023.
7. Robert Wood Johnson Foundation. Charting a course for an equity-centered data system. October 1, 2021. Available at: https://www.rwjf.org/en/insights/our-research/2021/10/charting-a-course-for-an-equity-centered-data-system.html. Accessed October 19, 2023.
8. Mittmann H, Heinrich J, Levi J. Accountable communities for health: what we are learning from recent evaluations. October 31, 2022. Available at: https://nam.edu/accountable-communities-for-health-what-we-are-learning-from-recent-evaluations/https://doi.org/10.31478/202210a. Accessed October 19, 2023.
9. de Guia S, Novais AP. Community trust and relationships: the key for strengthening public health systems. February 28, 2023. Available at: https://www.healthaffairs.org/content/forefront/community-trust-and-relationships-key-strengthening-public-health-systems. Accessed October 19, 2023.

Harnessing Telehealth: Improving Epidemic Prediction and Response

Gerardo Chowell, PhD, and Andrew Lawson, PhD

ABOUT THE AUTHORS

Gerardo Chowell is with the Department of Population Health Sciences, School of Public Health, Georgia State University, Atlanta. Andrew Lawson is with the Department of Public Health Sciences, Medical University of South Carolina, Charleston, and the Usher Institute, Centre for Population Health Sciences, Edinburgh Medical School, University of Edinburgh, Edinburgh, UK.

See also Haenchen et al., p. 218.

The coronavirus disease 2019 (COVID-19) pandemic has highlighted the need to develop robust and reliable forecasting tools to predict the course of epidemics and pandemics in near real time. Although data derived from traditional surveillance systems are the bedrock for tracking the impact of rapidly evolving infectious disease emergencies, harnessing novel data streams, such as those derived from telehealth platforms, has emerged as a critical strategy to fill this gap.[1]

Telehealth,[2] which saw unprecedented uptake because of social distancing measures and health care access challenges during the COVID-19 pandemic, generates vast amounts of data that can reflect real-time trends in symptom reporting, health care demand, and the efficacy of interventions. A thorough assessment of how telehealth data can be leveraged to enhance forecasting performance is crucial. Reliable forecasts can provide more granular insights into the spread and impact of infectious diseases, thus empowering public health leaders to make informed, timely decisions to allocate resources and implement interventions. In this issue of AJPH, Haenchen et al. (p. 218) have contributed to the ongoing research by examining and comparing the performance of statistical models for 14-day forecasts of COVID-19 cases and deaths. Their study distinguishes between models that exclusively utilize traditional data sources and those enhanced with telehealth data from a national telehealth provider serving 50 states and the District of Columbia. Their findings suggest that telehealth-based probable COVID-19 cases have the potential to improve short-term disease forecasts. This study should inspire subsequent analyses to understand the optimal methods for leveraging telehealth data in predictive modeling. In this article, we highlight issues relating to telehealth data privacy, accessibility, and representativeness and point out some considerations that should be taken into account in future forecasting studies to enhance their robustness and applicability.

The real-time application of telehealth data for predictive modeling presents significant privacy and security issues that must be carefully protected.[3] As these data streams often contain sensitive personal health information, they are subject to stringent data protection laws, such as the Health Insurance Portability and Accountability Act (HIPAA) in the United States. Ensuring that individual privacy is maintained is vital for preventing unauthorized data breaches. Additionally, the real-time requirement for forecasting exacerbates the challenge, as systems must be designed to allow instantaneous and secure data sharing. This poses a potential risk of increased vulnerability to cyberattacks because of the greater number of opportunities for unauthorized access. Continuous monitoring of data security practices, regular audits, and advanced cybersecurity measures can be implemented to mitigate these risks. Moreover, these measures must be transparent and maintain the trust of patients and health care providers without compromising the integrity and utility of the data for disease forecasting purposes.

As noted by Haenchen et al., telehealth coverage tends to be skewed toward working-age adults. Moreover, a study found that seniors, non-English speakers, and Black patients were more reliant on telephone than video for care during the COVID-19 pandemic.[4] Hence, the issue of data representativeness is crucial in the context of telehealth and its integration into epidemiological surveillance systems for disease modeling and forecasting. The data derived from telehealth services must reflect the diverse demographics and underlying health characteristics of the population under study to feed valuable data into models for disease prediction. However, systemic disparities in access to telehealth—influenced by factors such as socioeconomic status, health insurance coverage, age, and technology literacy—can lead to significant biases in the data, hindering their utility in public health decision-making and potentially exacerbating health inequalities. In addition, the bias introduced in telehealth access is exacerbated by asymptomatic transmission, which is not recorded. During the COVID-19 pandemic, estimates of asymptomatic transmission varied from 20% up to 50%,[5] so low ascertainment is a crucial factor in prediction accuracy. To address these issues, real-time data streams must be carefully evaluated for biases, and predictive models must be adjusted to account for these discrepancies.

Real-time accessibility of telehealth data is crucial for effective predictive modeling. Nevertheless, telehealth data are often owned by third parties, which limits timely data flow to researchers.[6] Moreover, integrating data from different providers may present technical challenges because of incompatible data systems and formats. In addition, different telehealth systems may capture trends at different levels of spatial resolution or focus on specific populations. These challenges will require efforts to develop robust interoperability standards, secure data-sharing agreements, and foster collaborations prioritizing high-quality, real-time telehealth data availability.

The study by Haenchen et al. provides a valuable contribution for using telehealth data in disease forecasting. However, several considerations should be taken into account in future research to enhance the robustness and applicability of forecasting methods. First, relying on a single data set may yield results that are not generally applicable; thus, it is crucial to test forecasting methods across multiple, varied data sets to establish generalizability. Second, performance metrics that account for the uncertainty in the predictions, such as the weighted interval score, should be employed for a more comprehensive assessment of performance. Finally, comparing the results of Haenchen et al. with alternative forecasting methods, such as those that account for spatial structure and underlying latent subepidemic processes, could yield more sophisticated insights into disease transmission dynamics.[7–9] In general, future forecasting studies should also aim to benchmark a variety of mathematical models and forecasting methods against a wide range of infectious diseases, considering different social contexts and geographical scales.[10,11] This comprehensive approach will help to create a standardized framework for assessing the efficacy of forecasting tools, ensuring that they are tested and validated across the broad spectrum of epidemiological scenarios.

Future research is essential to address the intricacies of data acquisition and integration and refine the methodologies that could unlock the full potential of telehealth data in strengthening epidemic forecasting tools. The analysis by Haenchen et al. stands as an illustrative case, indicating that data from telehealth platforms may be key to improving short-term predictions of disease spread, such as with COVID-19. While acknowledging the potential of telehealth data, we have also highlighted several challenges that must be addressed, including data representativeness, accessibility, and privacy. We hope this emerging work will spark further research and dialogue on optimizing telehealth data, not only for COVID-19 but across various infectious diseases, ultimately contributing to more effective disease prediction and management strategies. AJPH

CORRESPONDENCE

Correspondence should be sent to Gerardo Chowell, Georgia State University School of Public Health, 140 Decatur St SE, Atlanta, GA 30303. Reprints can be ordered at http://www.ajph.org by clicking the "Reprints" link.

PUBLICATION INFORMATION

Full Citation: Chowell G, Lawson A. Harnessing telehealth: improving epidemic prediction and response. *Am J Public Health*. 2024;114(2): 146–148.

Acceptance date: November 22, 2023.

DOI: https://doi.org/10.2105/AJPH.2023.307547

CONTRIBUTORS

Both authors contributed to the writing of the manuscript.

ACKNOWLEDGMENTS

G. Chowell acknowledges support from National Science Foundation (NSF) grant 2125246.

CONFLICTS OF INTEREST

The authors have no conflicts of interest to declare relating to the content of this article.

REFERENCES

1. Althouse BM, Scarpino SV, Meyers LA, et al. Enhancing disease surveillance with novel data streams: challenges and opportunities. *EPJ Data Sci*. 2015;4(1):17. https://doi.org/10.1140/epjds/s13688-015-0054-0
2. Tuckson RV, Edmunds M, Hodgkins ML. Telehealth. *N Engl J Med*. 2017;377(16):1585–1592. https://doi.org/10.1056/NEJMsr1503323
3. Hall JL, McGraw D. For telehealth to succeed, privacy and security risks must be identified and addressed. *Health Aff (Millwood)*. 2014;33(2): 216–221. https://doi.org/10.1377/hlthaff.2013.0997
4. Sachs JW, Graven P, Gold JA, Kassakian SZ. Disparities in telephone and video telehealth engagement during the COVID-19 pandemic. *JAMIA Open*. 2021;4(3):ooab056. https://doi.org/10.1093/jamiaopen/ooab056
5. Ma Q, Liu J, Liu Q, et al. Global percentage of asymptomatic SARS-CoV-2 infections among the tested population and individuals with confirmed COVID-19 diagnosis: a systematic review and meta-analysis. *JAMA Netw Open*. 2021;4(12): e2137257. https://doi.org/10.1001/jamanetworkopen.2021.37257
6. Kaplan B. Revisiting health information technology ethical, legal, and social issues and evaluation: telehealth/telemedicine and COVID-19. *Int J Med Inform*. 2020;143:104239. https://doi.org/10.1016/j.ijmedinf.2020.104239

7. Lawson AB. Evaluation of predictive capability of Bayesian spatio-temporal models for Covid-19 spread. *BMC Med Res Methodol.* 2023;23(1):182. https://doi.org/10.1186/s12874-023-01997-3
8. Lawson AB, Kim J. Bayesian space-time SIR modeling of Covid-19 in two US states during the 2020–2021 pandemic. *PLoS One.* 2022;17(12): e0278515. https://doi.org/10.1371/journal.pone.0278515
9. Chowell G, Dahal S, Tariq A, Roosa K, Hyman JM, Luo R. An ensemble n-sub-epidemic modeling framework for short-term forecasting epidemic trajectories: application to the COVID-19 pandemic in the USA. *PLOS Comput Biol.* 2022;18(10): e1010602. https://doi.org/10.1371/journal.pcbi.1010602
10. Bleichrodt A, Luo R, Kirpich A, Chowell G. Retrospective evaluation of short-term forecast performance of ensemble sub-epidemic frameworks and other time-series models: the 2022–2023 mpox outbreak across multiple geographical scales, July 14th, 2022, through February 26th, 2023. Preprint. *medRxiv.* 2023;2023.05.15.23289989. October 17, 2023. https://doi.org/10.1101/2023.05.15.23289989
11. Perry AG, Moore KM, Levesque LE, Pickett CWL, Korenberg MJ. A comparison of methods for forecasting emergency department visits for respiratory illness using telehealth Ontario calls. *Can J Public Health.* 2010;101(6):464–469. https://doi.org/10.1007/BF03403965

Tuberculosis in US Indigenous Communities: A Need for Public Health Prioritization

Lucia Cilloni, PhD, and David W. Dowdy, MD, PhD

ABOUT THE AUTHORS

The authors are with the Johns Hopkins Bloomberg School of Public Health, Johns Hopkins University, Baltimore, MD.

See also Springer et al., p. 226.

Indigenous communities continue to be confronted by health care challenges rooted in a history of colonization and forced displacement. This history is often reflected in less stable living conditions, fewer employment opportunities, lower income levels, and reduced access to food, water, and sanitation services. Geographic isolation, poverty, discrimination, and a lack of cultural understanding on the part of historical colonizers can create structural barriers to health care access among indigenous populations.[1] Although racial and ethnic health disparities are increasingly recognized as a major contributor to poor health outcomes in the United States,[2] the specific needs of indigenous communities are often underrepresented in efforts to address these disparities. As a result, members of indigenous communities can experience health outcomes that are often worse even than those of other racial and ethnic minorities (e.g., Black and Hispanic Americans).

One striking example of this structural neglect of indigenous populations is seen in incidence rates of tuberculosis (TB).[3] People identifying as American Indian/Alaska Native (AI/AN) or Native Hawaiian/Other Pacific Islander (NH/OPI) have a TB risk that is more than twice as high as non-Hispanic Black Americans and more than 10 times higher than that of White Americans. These estimates may, in fact, underrepresent the magnitude of the underlying disparities, as multiracial and Hispanic AI/AN individuals have been systematically excluded from corresponding data sets (see Springer et al., p. 226 in this issue of *AJPH*).

Furthermore, although TB incidence in these other US-born groups has been declining over the past decade, little progress has been made among AI/AN or NH/OPI populations, resulting in even greater disparities over time.[3] This higher prevalence of TB among indigenous populations is believed to reflect higher rates of ongoing transmission, meaning that interventions to control transmission (e.g., contact investigation) should be particularly effective in these communities.[4,5] Persistently high rates of TB in indigenous populations suggest that such interventions have not been implemented to their fullest potential.

The disproportionate burden of TB among indigenous communities has unfortunately been recognized for decades. More than 60 years ago, a tuberculin survey among Alaska Natives in the Yukon–Kuskokwim delta region indicated a latent TB infection (LTBI) prevalence above 75%, among the highest levels ever recorded.[6] This region also saw higher rates of TB mortality among indigenous populations than among White Alaskans, largely as a result of poor living conditions, lower economic means, and geographical isolation.[6] Intentional efforts to find people with TB and offer preventive treatment have dramatically reduced the burden of disease among these communities over time; such efforts have been successful because they have prioritized active engagement of, and ownership by, indigenous communities themselves.[6]

The systemic exclusion of indigenous communities from efforts to end TB in the United States is also reflected in the US Preventive Services Task Force recommendations to screen for LTBI in adults.[7] On one hand, the task force notes that certain racial and ethnic groups are disproportionately affected by TB. On the other hand, however, its explicit examples of populations at increased TB risk include only "persons who were born in, or are former residents of, countries with high TB prevalence and persons who live in, or have lived in, high-risk congregate settings (e.g., homeless shelters or correctional facilities)."[7] Thus, even though AI/AN and NH/OPI populations experience a similar burden of TB as people who were born outside the United States but entered early in life (e.g., by the age of 5 years[8]), the latter are far more likely to be screened for LTBI.

Expanding these recommendations to more explicitly include members of indigenous communities (as is done in Canada, for example[9]) would be a valuable first step. This should be

AJPH February 2024, Vol. 114, No. 2

followed by intentional efforts to partner with indigenous communities, empowering those communities to close this long-standing health disparity. Such efforts could include raising awareness of the risk of TB—and the availability of effective, short-course treatment options for LTBI—among community members and indigenous health providers and providing the resources (e.g., access to LTBI testing and treatment free of charge to individuals) necessary for indigenous community members to take charge of their own health.

The health inequities faced by indigenous populations are not specific to TB alone. As an example, indigenous populations face lower life expectancies (an estimated 11-year disparity in 2021 relative to non-Hispanic Whites and Native Americans) and have higher rates of diabetes, opioid and alcohol abuse, and depression, the latter three exacerbated further by the COVID-19 pandemic.[2,10] Again, these inequities are unfortunate legacies of colonialism, systemic racism, and intentional erasure, processes that continue to this day.

Fortunately, a number of programs that include and prioritize collaborative and inclusive practices have been successful in reducing the burden of disease in indigenous populations; lessons learned from these programs can also be applied to TB.[10] Indigenous-led programs such as the CheckUp Project and Peers4Wellness have facilitated research and outreach among indigenous women in Canada, in turn reducing the burden of HIV and hepatitis C virus.[10] Another example of an inclusive model is the "wise practices" approach, which promotes the inclusion of local culture, knowledge, and values into the design and implementation of health interventions.[11] Such interventions must take into account the heritage and priorities of each unique community.[11] If we are to effectively address the disproportionate burden of TB among indigenous communities in the United States, it is critical that models such as these be upheld and expanded, placing agency for improving health into the hands of indigenous people and communities themselves.[10]

In summary, despite growing recognition of racial and ethnic health disparities, indigenous communities in the United States still face pervasive health care challenges, and their unique needs often remain overlooked. Tuberculosis serves as an important example, with indigenous populations experiencing significantly higher incidence rates than other racial and ethnic groups, indicating a systemic failure in implementing effective interventions. Fortunately, the excess burden of TB among indigenous communities is an addressable problem with a historical precedent of success through efforts that emphasize collaboration and inclusivity and that empower communities. These efforts should be supplemented with structural solutions including more representative data reporting, updated guidelines for TB prevention, and provision of the resources necessary to effectively implement those guidelines. TB can be ended in American indigenous populations as effectively as it can among White Americans; failure to close this disparity in the coming five to 10 years will be a stain on the US public health system as a whole. AJPH

CORRESPONDENCE

Correspondence should be sent to David W. Dowdy, MD, PhD, 615 N Wolfe St, W1513A, Baltimore, MD 21205 (e-mail: ddowdy1@jhmi.edu). Reprints can be ordered at http://www.ajph.org by clicking the "Reprints" link.

PUBLICATION INFORMATION

Full Citation: Cilloni L, Dowdy DW. Tuberculosis in US indigenous communities: a need for public health prioritization. *Am J Public Health*. 2024; 114(2):149–151.

Acceptance Date: November 27, 2023.

DOI: https://10.2105/AJPH.2023.307544

CONTRIBUTORS

L. Cilloni wrote the initial draft. D.W. Dowdy revised the article substantially for intellectual content. Both authors made subsequent revisions.

CONFLICTS OF INTEREST

The authors have no conflicts of interest to declare.

REFERENCES

1. United Nations Economic and Social Affairs. State of the world's indigenous peoples: indigenous peoples' access to health services. Available at: https://www.un.org/development/desa/indigenouspeoples/publications/state-of-the-worlds-indigenous-peoples.html. Accessed November 12, 2023.
2. Health, United States, 2015: *With Special Feature on Racial and Ethnic Health Disparities.* Hyattsville, MD: National Center for Health Statistics; 2016.
3. Centers for Disease Control and Prevention. Tuberculosis in the United States slide set. Available at: https://www.cdc.gov/tb/statistics/surv/surv2022/default.htm. Accessed November 12, 2023.
4. Springer YP, Kammerer JS, Silk BJ, Langer AJ. Tuberculosis in indigenous persons—United States, 2009–2019. *J Racial Ethn Health Disparities.* 2022;9(5):1750–1764. https://doi.org/10.1007/s40615-021-01112-6
5. Centers for Disease Control and Prevention. Tuberculosis outbreak on an American Indian reservation—Montana, 2000–2001. *MMWR Morb Mortal Wkly Rep.* 2002;51(11):232–234.
6. Comstock GW, Philip RN. Decline of the tuberculosis epidemic in Alaska. *Public Health Rep (1896).* 1961;76(1):19–24.
7. US Preventive Services Task Force. Latent tuberculosis infection in adults. Available at: https://www.uspreventiveservicestaskforce.org/uspstf/recommendation/latent-tuberculosis-infection-screening. Accessed November 12, 2023.
8. Hill AN, Cohen T, Salomon JA, Menzies NA. High-resolution estimates of tuberculosis incidence

among non-US-born persons residing in the United States, 2000–2016. *Epidemics*. 2020; 33:100419. https://doi.org/10.1016/j.epidem.2020.100419

9. Government of Canada. Tuberculosis surveillance and screening in selected high-risk populations. Available at: https://www.canada.ca/en/public-health/services/infectious-diseases/canadian-tuberculosis-standards-7th-edition/edition-9.html. Accessed November 12, 2023.

10. Lee NR, King A, Vigil D, et al. Infectious diseases in indigenous populations in North America: learning from the past to create a more equitable future. *Lancet Infect Dis*. 2023;23(10): e431–e444. https://doi.org/10.1016/S1473-3099(23)00190-1

11. Wesley-Esquimaux C, Calliou B. Best practices in Aboriginal community development: a literature review and wise practices approach. Available at: https://communities4families.ca/wp-content/uploads/2014/08/Aboriginal-Community-Development.pdf. Accessed November 12, 2023.

Opportunities for Increasing Access to Person-Centered Abortion Care Through Telehealth

Erica Munson, MPH, and Kelli S. Hall, PhD

ABOUT THE AUTHORS

Erica Munson and Kelli S. Hall are with the Heilbrunn Department of Population and Family Health, Mailman School of Public Health, Columbia University, New York, NY.

See also Koenig et al., p. 241.

As provision of in-clinic abortion becomes increasingly restricted in the United States, telehealth medication abortion has great potential to fill access gaps as an alternative mode of care delivery.[1] Telehealth abortion has the potential to expand abortion access to an additional 3.5 million people of reproductive age in the United States.[2] A person-centered approach should be front and center in efforts to guide adaptation, implementation, and sustainability of telehealth abortion care.

Although the Food and Drug Administration has modified the risk evaluation and mitigation strategies to allow for mail-delivery medication abortion, the overturning of *Roe v Wade* in the *Dobbs v Jackson Women's Health Organization* court case has given states the power to implement policies that differentially limit provision of abortion services through telehealth across the country. State laws restricting telehealth abortion disproportionately occur in locations where nonlegislative barriers to abortion are already prevalent and socially disadvantaged populations suffer high rates of adverse sexual and reproductive and maternal health outcomes; these include those residing in rural areas, low resource communities, racially and ethnically minoritized groups, and people living in poverty.[3,4]

At the same time, the proliferation of state-level abortion laws following the *Dobbs v Jackson* decision has further shaped an environment of unmet need for comprehensive facility-based services that offer high-quality, in-person care and an increased need for access through other delivery modes, including telehealth[5,6]; this may be especially true in states with the most restrictive policy climates.[7]

Currently, 14 states have a near-total ban on abortion in effect and 15 states restrict access to medication abortion; five of these states require the patient to have an in-person visit with a physician, effectively prohibiting telehealth abortion.[8] Self-managed abortion (defined as abortion that takes place outside of the formal health care setting), when provided through online telemedicine may provide similar opportunities to telehealth medication abortion for persons living in states with telehealth abortion restrictions. For example, self-managed abortion through the organization Aid Access, operating outside the US health care setting in all 50 states, provides mail-delivery medication abortion through an online platform and has been found to be effective, acceptable to users, and to have a very low rate of serious adverse outcomes.[1] Although self-managed abortion is not illegal in the majority of US states, it can still hold legal risks, including being reported and investigated after postabortion care is sought.[1,9] To combat the legal risks of abortion, some states have enacted shield laws to protect persons crossing state lines to receive abortion care. Interstate shield laws, which have been enacted primarily in the Northeast and the West, limit criminal prosecution or civil enforcement of abortion restrictions across state lines.[9] Shield laws could provide an access avenue for persons residing in legally restrictive states who desire telehealth medication abortion services.

Other well-documented barriers to abortion access include provider shortages and care deserts outside of urban centers, long travel distances, costs, child care support or the need to take time off work, and other logistical needs.[4,10] In states where it is not legally banned, telehealth abortion can mitigate these factors.[4,10] Importantly, studies have shown that telehealth abortion provision does not significantly increase patients' time from first contact with the clinic to medication ingestion, or increase pregnancy duration at medication ingestion.[11] Additionally, there is evidence of a positive association between distance to the nearest clinic and desire for telehealth services.[12] One qualitative study consisting of semistructured interviews

AJPH February 2024, Vol. 114, No. 2

with individuals who received mail-delivery medication abortion found that going to a clinic was so burdensome for some participants that they would not have otherwise been able to get an abortion.[13] These participants cited travel, clinic availability, logistics, and costs as burdens associated with receiving an in-clinic abortion and felt that direct-to-patient telemedicine abortion was more convenient and accessible.[13] Although geographic location is an important indicator of need for alternative abortion care models, some people choose telehealth over an equidistant clinic option, suggesting that a myriad of factors influence preferences for and the values placed on different service delivery models, which then affect health decision-making and care-seeking behaviors.[10]

ACCEPTABILITY OF TELEHEALTH ABORTION

In this issue of the *American Journal of Public Health*, Koenig et al. (p. 241) analyzed secondary data from 1600 telehealth abortion patients surveyed between June 2021 and January 2022 in the California Home Abortion by Telehealth Study. The authors report remarkable positive estimates for telehealth abortion services across a series of person-centered indicators, including acceptability and satisfaction. Nearly all of those surveyed (89%) were satisfied with the care they received and felt that telehealth was the right decision (96%).

Drivers of satisfaction with telehealth abortion may relate to patients' ability to take the pills in the privacy, comfort, and convenience of their own home,[13] thus ensuring access for those who do not have the time or resources to see a provider in-person[10] and those who may experience provider and health facility mistrust, stigma, or discrimination.[7]

Koenig et al.'s study advances this prior work by assessing patient acceptability across synchronous and asynchronous care settings—which have been understudied dimensions of health services research on abortion. The authors gathered data from three different clinics, one of which used synchronous communication via phone or video call, whereas the other two screened patients using an online consultation form and followed up with asynchronous communication via secure written messages. Both service delivery modes were correlated with high levels of patient satisfaction, trust, and a feeling that telehealth was the right choice. These findings provide new insights on the implications for the adaptability, implementation, and sustainability of telehealth abortion in ways that meet the desires and values of patients across diverse settings and populations that telehealth has potential to reach. As Koenig et al. note, policies that protect patients' ability to access both synchronous and asynchronous modes of care and providers' and health systems' ability to support them are urgently warranted in the United States.

LOOKING BEYOND ACCESS AND ACCEPTABILITY

Person-centered care has been defined by the Institute of Medicine as crucial to quality health care,[14] and inclusive of respectful care that accounts for patients' cultural and other values, preferences, and needs.[14] Similarly, the World Health Organization's Abortion Care Guideline offers a key human rights consideration on respectful care within service-delivery models, stating that "Sexual and reproductive health services must be available, accessible, affordable, acceptable and of good quality. This means that delivery of services must be respectful of the culture of individuals, minorities, peoples and communities, and sensitive to gender, age, disability, sexual diversity and life-cycle requirements."[15]

Koenig et al.'s study highlights that successful strategies to ensure accessible and acceptable abortion care through telehealth require policy and health systems changes targeting the other essential dimensions of person-centeredness. For example, payor reform, including Medicaid expansion and private insurance coverage, increased capacity to provide services that are culturally congruent and offered in multiple languages, and care models that protect minors' access to confidential care and meet the needs of older reproductive age groups are necessary considerations for available, affordable, and quality care. Further inequities exist in a digital divide, where neighborhoods predominately populated by people of color lack Internet access and other technology resources compared with wealthier, White neighborhoods.[3] One study comparing telehealth engagement and modality use found that non-English speakers, Black patients, and those insured by Medicaid or Medicare were more likely to use telephone than video compared with other telehealth users.[3] Efforts to address this digital divide can expand access to Internet and other technology resources and remove barriers to digital access—for example, through policies that increase broadband connectivity, affordability, and device utilization, especially for the most disadvantaged groups and underserved settings.[3]

Other respectful-care considerations include ensuring that service delivery modes, like synchronous and asynchronous telehealth care, can be adapted in ways that are equitable in meeting the needs of individuals' gender identity, age, disability status, sexual orientation, and life-course stage.[15] Although Koenig et al.'s study includes one of the most geographically diverse samples of telehealth abortion patients in the United States of which we are aware, the authors recognize that the study participants were disproportionately White (53%), older, and more financially secure than the national population of abortion patients. Additional research should prioritize the voices and lived experiences of patients, providers, and communities who represent a broad range of racial and ethnic, socioeconomic, and geographic backgrounds.

CONCLUSIONS

Telehealth abortion offers a timely model of person-centered reproductive health care in the United States. Multilevel strategies that center a health equity and human rights framework will be central to guiding effective adaptation, implementation, and sustainability of telehealth abortion in ways that ensure not only access and acceptability, but affordable, respectful, quality, and equitable care. Ultimately, in our complex post-*Roe* landscape, telehealth abortion holds great promise for reducing health and health care disparities and improving the well-being of diverse patients and communities across the country.[3] AJPH

CORRESPONDENCE

Correspondence should be sent to Erica Munson, 239 East 84th St, New York, NY 10028 (e-mail: ericamackenzie@berkeley.edu). Reprints can be ordered at http://www.ajph.org by clicking the "Reprints" link.

PUBLICATION INFORMATION

Full Citation: Munson E, Hall KS. Opportunities for increasing access to person-centered abortion care through telehealth. *Am J Public Health*. 2024;114(2):152–154.

Acceptance Date: November 26, 2023.

DOI: https://doi.org/10.2105/AJPH.2023.307541

CONTRIBUTORS

E. Munson and K. S. Hall conceptualized and refined the focus of the article. E. Munson conducted the literature review and wrote the first draft, with substantive contributions from K. S. Hall. Both authors contributed to the revisioning and finalization of the article.

CONFLICTS OF INTEREST

The authors have no conflicts of interest to disclose.

REFERENCES

1. Aiken ARA, Romanova EP, Morber JR, Gomperts R. Safety and effectiveness of self-managed medication abortion provided using online telemedicine in the United States: a population based study. *Lancet Reg Health Am.* 2022;10:100200. https://doi.org/10.1016/j.lana.2022.100200
2. Seymour JW, Thompson TA, Milechin D, Wise LA, Rudolph AE. Potential impact of telemedicine for medication abortion policy and programming changes on abortion accessibility in the United States. *Am J Public Health.* 2022;112(8):1202–1211. https://doi.org/10.2105/AJPH.2022.306876
3. Thompson TA, Northcraft D, Carrión F. Addressing structural inequities, a necessary step toward ensuring equitable access to telehealth for medication abortion care during and post COVID-19. *Front Glob Womens Health.* 2022; 3:805767. https://doi.org/10.3389/fgwh.2022.805767
4. Clure C, Sheeder J, Teal S, Cohen R. Telemedicine to improve reproductive health care for rural Coloradans: perceptions of interest and access. *J Rural Health.* 2023;39(1):172–178. https://doi.org/10.1111/jrh.12697
5. Aiken ARA, Starling JE, Scott JG, Gomperts R. Requests for self-managed medication abortion provided using online telemedicine in 30 US states before and after the Dobbs v Jackson Women's Health Organization Decision. *JAMA.* 2022;328(17):1768–1770. https://doi.org/10.1001/jama.2022.18865
6. Aiken ARA, Starling JE, Scott JG, Gomperts R. Association of Texas Senate Bill 8 with requests for self-managed medication abortion. *JAMA Netw Open.* 2022;5(2):e221122. https://doi.org/10.1001/jamanetworkopen.2022.1122
7. Rivlin K, Brenner-Levoy J, Odum T, et al. Provider mistrust and telemedicine abortion care preferences among patients in Ohio, West Virginia, and Kentucky. *Telemed J E Health.* 2023;29(3):414-424. https://doi.org/10.1089/tmj.2022.0101
8. Guttmacher Institute. Medication abortion. February 6, 2023. Available at: https://www.guttmacher.org/state-policy/explore/medication-abortion. Accessed February 27, 2023.
9. Ghorashi A, Baumle D. Legal and health risks of abortion criminalization: state policy responses in the immediate aftermath of Dobbs. *J Law Health.* 2023;37(1):6, 17–18.
10. Beardsworth KM, Doshi U, Raymond E, Baldwin MK. Miles and days until medical abortion via TelAbortion versus clinic in Oregon and Washington, USA. *BMJ Sex Reprod Health.* 2022;48(e1): e38–e43. https://doi.org/10.1136/bmjsrh-2020-200972
11. Koenig LR, Raymond EG, Gold M, et al. Mailing abortion pills does not delay care: a cohort study comparing mailed to in-person dispensing of abortion medications in the United States. *Contraception.* 2023;121:109962. https://doi.org/10.1016/j.contraception.2023.109962
12. Aiken ARA, Starling JE, Gomperts R. Factors associated with use of an online telemedicine service to access self-managed medical abortion in the US. *JAMA Netw Open.* 2021;4(5):e2111852. https://doi.org/10.1001/jamanetworkopen.2021.11852
13. Kerestes C, Delafield R, Elia J, Chong E, Kaneshiro B, Soon R. "It was close enough, but it wasn't close enough": a qualitative exploration of the impact of direct-to-patient telemedicine abortion on access to abortion care. *Contraception.* 2021; 104(1):67–72. https://doi.org/10.1016/j.contraception.2021.04.028
14. Tzelepis F, Sanson-Fisher RW, Zucca AC, Fradgley EA. Measuring the quality of patient-centered care: why patient-reported measures are critical to reliable assessment. *Patient Prefer Adherence.* 2015;9:831–835. https://doi.org/10.2147/PPA.S81975
15. World Health Organization. Abortion care guideline. Available at: https://www.who.int/publications-detail-redirect/9789240039483. Accessed September 23, 2023.

Vaccine Hesitancy, Pharmaceutical Marketing, and Mistrusted Messengers

James Colgrove, PhD, MPH

ABOUT THE AUTHOR

James Colgrove is with the Center for the History and Ethics of Public Health, Department of Sociomedical Sciences, Mailman School of Public Health, Columbia University, New York, NY.

See also Lanzarotta, p. 193.

In this issue of *AJPH*, Lanzarotta (p. 193) examines how manufacturers of the smallpox vaccine sought to assuage doubts about their product during the 19th century, when the risks of vaccine-adverse events were far greater than they are today. Her cogent historical analysis highlights Americans' shifting attitudes toward pharmaceutical products, the ways that the alleged and actual risks of vaccination fostered hesitancy, and the enduring relationship between public trust in drug companies and the acceptance or rejection of vaccines. Americans have looked with optimism on the prospects that new diagnostics, vaccines, and treatments would extend life and improve its quality; at the same time, they have also questioned the motives and integrity of pharmaceutical companies and the effects of the profit motive on drug producers' behavior. Historically and in the present day, these concerns have undermined vaccine acceptance and have fueled both hesitancy and active opposition and resistance.

Pharmaceutical companies began to assume their modern form in the early 20th century on the heels of the scientific breakthroughs of the bacteriological revolution. They developed more sophisticated methods of studying, producing, and marketing drugs and employed larger staffs with formal training in medicine and bacteriology.[1] As Lanzarotta notes, this new model was a significant change from the small-scale, mostly unregulated "farms" where the smallpox vaccine had been propagated in cattle during the 19th century.

This transformation provided a basis for drug companies to credibly argue that vaccination was a safe and effective procedure backed by the best science. However, these developments were also accompanied by heightened scrutiny and criticism of the medical research establishment. Negative publicity surrounded drug studies in which doctors conducted human participants research on populations who lacked the ability to give their informed consent, such as orphans, people with mental disabilities, incarcerated people, and gravely ill hospital patients.[2]

Critics of vaccination seized on these incidents and accused pharmaceutical companies of callousness and greed. In their view, drug makers' profit-seeking goals presented an irreconcilable conflict of interest with whatever health-promoting mission they professed. Vaccine critics allied with related political movements such as antivivisection activism, which fought against the use of laboratory animals to test new treatments and cures and which argued, with justification, that animal research would lead to unethical experimentation on vulnerable humans. Antivaccination political activism was widespread in the early 20th century, with legislative battles over issues such as vaccination mandates and the compulsory medical inspection of schoolchildren, which critics saw as medical elites' coercive intrusions into spheres of private decision-making that belonged to families.[3] Vaccine hesitancy reflected broader concerns about the character and intentions of scientific authorities.

By the mid-20th century, misgivings about the dark side of scientific progress had largely faded amid a dazzling parade of biomedical advances. The post-WWII period was the era of "miracle cures" and "wonder drugs," with breakthroughs in treatments for hypertension, mental illness, hemophilia, tuberculosis, arthritis, and many other conditions. This period was the high-water mark of Americans' acclaim for and trust in pharmaceutical products. Although politicians and policymakers raised concerns about drug costs and safety, the industry successfully resisted efforts to regulate it.[4] Laboratory scientists were cultural heroes, their achievements covered in admiring news stories that were often engineered, and sometimes ghostwritten, by the pharmaceutical companies' sophisticated public relations outfits.[5]

Not coincidentally, antivaccination sentiment remained a fringe phenomenon in this era, barely noted in mainstream media coverage. When the Salk polio vaccine was licensed in 1955, arguably the crowning achievement in 20th-century vaccine development, there were virtually no concerns raised about its safety, even after the infamous "Cutter incident," in which contaminated lots of the vaccine caused dozens of cases of paralytic polio and at least five deaths.[6]

Today, pharma no longer enjoys such respect and acclaim. A 2023 survey showed that public opinion of the pharmaceutical industry is at its lowest level in decades, with only 18% of Americans holding a positive view and 60% holding a negative view.[7] A range of ethical controversies and political scandals have taken a toll on the industry's standing, including failure to disclose clinical trial results, illegal off-label marketing, overcharging Medicaid and Medicare, engineering the overprescribing of opioid painkillers, and various forms of profiteering that have led to the United States paying the highest drug prices in the world.

All these actions have provided ample fodder for vaccine skeptics. The Web sites of prominent antivaccination organizations, such as the National Vaccine Information Center and Robert Kennedy Jr's Children's Health Defense, paint a picture of the pharmaceutical industry as a malign cabal in league with government agencies and nongovernmental organizations, such as the Gates Foundation. This rhetoric, reflecting deep-seated mistrust of medical and scientific elites, echoes the claims of vaccine skeptics of a century ago.

In stark contrast to the mid–20th-century media landscape in which they cultivated their favorable image, pharmaceutical companies are no longer able to control the narrative about their activities and accomplishments. Distortions and falsehoods about vaccination circulate unchecked across social media platforms amid what the World Health Organization has termed an "infodemic." What give these claims credibility are actual instances in which pharmaceutical companies have engaged in illegal or unethical behavior. Many vaccine-skeptical arguments are built around a kernel of truth: that pharmaceutical companies, historically and in the present day, have sometimes engaged in negligent or unethical practices that have harmed patients.

Vaccine hesitancy is complex and has varied roots, including devotion to "natural" or alternative healing systems and mistrust in established sources of medical and public health authority. Although the poor reputation of the pharmaceutical industry may not be the most significant factor motivating vaccine hesitancy, it is clearly one of the drivers for many people.[8] The effect of this was apparent during the COVID-19 pandemic, when attitudes toward pharmaceutical companies, and the medical establishment more broadly, predicted people's intentions to receive newly approved COVID-19 vaccines.[9]

A widely recognized strategy for increasing vaccine confidence is the use of trusted messengers: individuals and organizations that can effectively convey provaccine messages because they enjoy high levels of public trust.[10] Lanzarotta rightly emphasizes the important role that trust plays in efforts to increase vaccine acceptance, and she argues that maintaining trust in vaccines in the 21st century will require "deft marketing and concerted efforts to educate the public" (p. 200). Although effective persuasion and education will no doubt be necessary, they will not be sufficient. No matter how clearly communicated the science underlying vaccination is, and how skillfully new vaccines are marketed, hesitancy will be difficult to address if the pharmaceutical industry continues to engage in actions that sow mistrust in its integrity and motives.

As the anthropologist Heidi Larson has argued, vaccine hesitancy is not so much a misinformation problem as it is a trust problem.[11] What is needed is not simply better marketing of vaccines; it is more trustworthy behavior on the part of the companies that make them. Rigorous adherence to legal and ethical guidelines and meaningful reforms to address drug cost and access will not be a panacea for building confidence in vaccines, but they are an excellent place to start. AJPH

CORRESPONDENCE

Correspondence should be sent to James Colgrove, Columbia Mailman School of Public Health, 722 West 168th St, New York, NY 10032 (e-mail: jc988@columbia.edu). Reprints can be ordered at http://www.ajph.org by clicking the "Reprints" link.

PUBLICATION INFORMATION

Full Citation: Colgrove J. Vaccine hesitancy, pharmaceutical marketing, and mistrusted messengers. *Am J Public Health*. 2024;114(2):155–157.

Acceptance Date: November 22, 2023.

DOI: https://doi.org/10.2105/AJPH.2023.307546

ACKNOWLEDGMENTS

The author thanks Robert Sember for comments on an earlier draft of this editorial.

CONFLICTS OF INTEREST

The author has no conflicts of interest to report.

REFERENCES

1. Galambos L, Sewell JE. *Networks of Innovation: Vaccine Development at Merck, Sharp & Dohme, and Mulford, 1895–1995*. Cambridge, UK: Cambridge University Press; 1995.
2. Lederer S. *Subjected to Science: Human Experimentation in America Before the Second World War*. Baltimore, MD: Johns Hopkins University Press; 1995.
3. Colgrove J. "Science in a democracy": the contested status of vaccination in the Progressive Era and the 1920s. *Isis*. 2005;96(2):167–191. https://doi.org/10.1086/431531
4. Tobbell DA. *Pills, Power, and Policy: The Struggle for Drug Reform in Cold War America and Its Consequences*. Berkeley, CA: University of California Press; 2012.

5. Greene JA, Herzberg D. Hidden in plain sight: marketing prescription drugs to consumers in the twentieth century. *Am J Public Health*. 2010;100(5):793–803. https://doi.org/10.2105/AJPH.2009.181255
6. Colgrove J. *State of Immunity: The Politics of Vaccination in Twentieth-Century America*. Berkeley, CA: University of California Press; 2006.
7. Saad L. Retail, pharmaceutical industries slip in public esteem. September 13, 2023. Available at: https://news.gallup.com/poll/510641/retail-pharmaceutical-industries-slip-public-esteem.aspx. Accessed October 31, 2023.
8. Lyman S. Pharma's tarnished reputation helps fuel the anti-vaccine movement. *STAT News*. February 26, 2019. Available at: https://www.statnews.com/2019/02/26/anti-vaccine-movement-pharma-tarnished-reputation. Accessed October 31, 2023.
9. Liu S, Chu H. Examining the direct and indirect effects of trust in motivating COVID-19 vaccine uptake. *Patient Educ Couns*. 2022;105(7):2096–2102. https://doi.org/10.1016/j.pec.2022.02.009
10. Shen AK, Browne S, Srivastava T, et al. Trusted messengers and trusted messages: the role for community-based organizations in promoting COVID-19 and routine immunizations. *Vaccine*. 2023;41(12):1994–2002. https://doi.org/10.1016/j.vaccine.2023.02.045
11. Larson HJ. *Stuck: How Vaccine Rumors Start—And Why They Don't Go Away*. New York, NY: Oxford University Press; 2020.

Adolescent Mental Health and Well-Being: A Public Health of Consequence, February 2024

Farzana Kapadia, PhD, MPH

ABOUT THE AUTHOR

Farzana Kapadia is the deputy editor of AJPH *and a professor of epidemiology at the School of Global Public Health, New York University, New York.*

Based on 2021 Centers for Disease Control and Prevention (CDC) data, more than 30% of US adolescents experienced poor mental health during the COVID-19 pandemic. Although availability of recent global data is limited, according to data collected as part of the Institute of Health Metric's 2019 Global Burden of Disease study, one of seven adolescents aged 10 to 19 years experienced a mental health condition worldwide (https://ghdx.healthdata.org). Depression, anxiety, and behavioral disorders account for the majority of adolescents' mental health burden and can negatively influence individual as well as collective health and well-being during this crucial period of development. Yet, implementation of effective policies and programs to prevent mental health burdens and to support those experiencing mental health conditions is uneven at best and wholly absent at worst. In addition, suicide is the fourth leading cause of death among adolescents and young adults aged 15 to 29 years worldwide. What these overall prevalence estimates mask are variations across countries, particularly variations driven by differences in data quality, availability of treatment services, and importantly, knowledge about mental health burdens and stigma associated with mental health illness.

Moreover, as we emerge from the social and physical distancing required during the COVID-19 pandemic, we also emerge into an era when the social isolation experienced by adolescents during the pandemic is compounded by growing fears and anxieties. Experiencing and even observing the growing burden of political, social, economic, and environmental adversities—such as an increasing number of political and military conflicts worldwide, forced migration, gun violence, restrictions on sexual and reproductive rights, increasing homophobia and transphobia, greater economic instability, and worsening climate crises—are strong social and structural drivers of mental health burdens among adolescents. Among adolescent girls of color and those who identify as gay, lesbian, bisexual, transgender, queer, and nonbinary, these adversities can be exacerbated by experiences of racism, discrimination, stigma, bullying, and adverse childhood events that amplify their risk of experiencing mental health burdens.

In this Public Health of Consequence, we focus on recent findings published in *AJPH* describing difficulties in accurately, appropriately, and consistently measuring mental health burdens among adolescents globally and highlight current efforts to provide more appropriate diagnostic tools for adolescents. Furthermore, we highlight sociocultural frameworks more relevant for adolescents as well as culturally tailored and age-appropriate interventions that may be effective at reducing or alleviating the harms associated with mental health burdens. Recognizing the importance of the social, political, and environmental shocks that adolescents are facing and navigating will allow public health practitioners to increase access to effective treatment and support services as well as prevention programs for those most vulnerable.

ESTIMATING MENTAL HEALTH BURDENS

Liu et al. used data from the 2022 Household Pulse Survey, fielded by the US Census Bureau, to provide estimates of parent-reported mental health symptoms among adolescents aged 18 years and younger.[1] Their findings, although based on parental report, indicate that 34.5% of adolescents experienced a mental health symptom (e.g., "feel anxious or clingy" or "feel very sad or depressed") in the past four weeks. Although these data are derived from parental reporting and are subject to information bias and also reflect a very short time frame (the previous four weeks), they are comparable to estimates obtained in the CDC's Adolescent Behaviors and Experiences Survey. These comparable estimates may suggest that we can rely on parental reporting to estimate adolescent mental health burden. However, proxy (e.g., parent) responses should be employed with caution. In addition, the types of measures used and time frames ascertained will affect the estimates of mental health burdens in adolescents. What these findings do call for is the consistent use of validated diagnostic measures in all population-based surveys that ascertain data on adolescent mental health, as the use of symptom-based scales in population-based surveys are unlikely to provide accurate estimates of true mental health burdens.

In addition, the development and use of consistent diagnostic measures of mental health burden in adolescents living in low- and middle-income countries (LMICs) face further challenges. Specifically, ensuring their cultural and linguistic appropriateness as well as their clinical relevance is required for diagnostic accuracy. The need for appropriate diagnostic tools cannot continue to be ignored given the growing burden of mental health conditions worldwide. To this point, a part of the Global Early Adolescent Study (https://www.geastudy.org), the National Adolescent Mental Health Surveys (NAMHS) serves as an example of a successful model of developing and implementing mental health assessment among adolescents in three distinct LMICs: Kenya, Vietnam, and Indonesia (https://bit.ly/3uoZhQV).

INTERVENTIONS THAT MEET ADOLESCENT NEEDS

Beyond accurate diagnostic tools for adolescent mental health burdens, the public health community need to ensure community engagement and buy-in as well as mental health service delivery capacity building to meet the mental health needs of adolescents. Recognizing that untreated mental health needs among adolescents are significant drivers of mental and physical health burdens in adulthood, particularly for minority adolescents, Hampton-Anderson et al. posit a sociocultural conceptual framework for reducing the disparities in mental health treatment utilization among Black adolescents.[2] The three standards of practice outlined here—using a sociocultural framework, exercising flexibility in one's assigned role, and understanding and incorporating culturally specific strengths and protective factors into care—echo those employed in the NAMHS. These similarities highlight how accurate and meaningful data should be collected as well as how policy and programmatic efforts can and should be informed to reduce mental health burdens among adolescents.

Given the significance of economic instability as a driver of mental and physical health burdens among adolescents in LMICs, Ssewamala et al. report on the Suubi4her study, a cluster-randomized controlled trial conducted across 47 public secondary schools in central Uganda.[3] Their findings provide evidence that conditional cash transfer can serve as a powerful economic empowerment tool for adolescents that can improve mental health outcomes.

NO HEALTH WITHOUT MENTAL HEALTH

Over the past decade, our global community has faced a growing number of shocks. As these challenges persist into the future, their impact on the mental health and well-being of adolescents cannot be ignored. Consistent and accurate measurement tools that allow researchers and advocates to understand the extent of mental health burdens as well as how social, political, and economic upheavals and climate crises drive these burdens is critical. With such information, we can continue the work of developing and testing interventions that disrupt the sociostructural drivers of poor mental health. As noted in the World Health Organization's World Mental Health Report, to strengthen policies and improve prevention programs as well as access to mental health treatment that improve the mental health of adolescents, we need "all stakeholders to work together to deepen the value and commitment given to mental health, reshape the environments that influence mental health, and strengthen the systems that care for mental health" (https://bit.ly/3GNfZMD). AJPH

CORRESPONDENCE

Correspondence should be sent to Farzana Kapadia, PhD, MPH, New York University, School of Global Public Health, 708 Broadway, Room 729, New York, NY 10003 (e-mail: farzana.kapadia@nyu.edu). Reprints can be ordered at http://www.ajph.org by clicking the "Reprints" link.

PUBLICATION INFORMATION

Full Citation: Kapadia F. Adolescent mental health and well-being: a Public Health of Consequence, February 2024. *Am J Public Health*. 2024;114(2): 158–160.

Acceptance Date: November 22, 2023.

DOI: https://doi.org/10.2105/AJPH.2023.307543

CONFLICTS OF INTEREST

The author has no conflicts of interest to disclose.

REFERENCES

1. Liu J, Zhou Z, Cheng X, Vangeepuram N. Geographic and sociodemographic variations in prevalence of mental health symptoms among US youths, 2022. *Am J Public Health*. 2023;113(10): 1116–1119. https://doi.org/10.2105/AJPH.2023.307355
2. Hampton-Anderson JN, Novacek DM, Zhen-Duan J, Latimer S, Perry T, Renard D. Redefining the role of public health professionals serving Black youths seeking mental health care: implications for training and mentoring. *Am J Public Health*. 2023;113(suppl 2):S140–S148. https://doi.org/10.2105/AJPH.2022.307194
3. Ssewamala FM, Brathwaite R, Neilands TB. Economic empowerment, HIV risk behavior, and mental health among school-going adolescent girls in Uganda: longitudinal cluster-randomized controlled trial, 2017–2022. *Am J Public Health*. 2023;113(3):306–315. https://doi.org/10.2105/AJPH.2022.307169

The Public Health Crisis State of Transgender Health Care and Policy

Arjee Javellana Restar, PhD, MPH, Eric K. Layland, PhD, Bee Davis, MS, Hale Thompson, PhD, and Carl Streed Jr, MD, MPH

ABOUT THE AUTHORS

Arjee Javellana Restar is with the departments of Epidemiology and Health Systems and Population Health, School of Public Health, University of Washington, Seattle, as well as the Department of Social and Behavioral Sciences, Yale University, New Haven, CT. Eric K. Layland is with the Department of Human Development and Family Sciences, University of Delaware, Newark. Bee Davis is with the Digital Forensics, Brown University, Providence, RI. Hale Thompson is with Howard Brown Health, Chicago, IL. Carl Streed Jr is with the Section of General Internal Medicine, Boston University Chobanian and Avedisian School of Medicine, and the GenderCare Center, Boston Medical Center, Boston, MA.

The rise of antitransgender legislation in the United States[1] has reached unprecedented levels. At the time of writing (October 2023), there were 574 bill proposals explicitly directed at transgender populations in 49 US states, of which 83 have been signed into law.[1] These bills aim to restrict the rights and freedoms of transgender persons, particularly children and adolescents, in areas of health care and society such as employment, education, sports, and public facilities, effectively excluding transgender persons from participating in civic life.

HEALTH IMPACTS OF ANTITRANSGENDER LEGISLATION

For instance, according to the Transgender Legislation Tracker,[2] of the 83 laws passed, 22 were specific to restricting access to and provision of health care (e.g., making medically endorsed best practices of gender-affirming care to minors a felony crime), 19 were aimed at education restrictions (e.g., use of pronouns, updating gender marker and name in school records, undermining the privacy of transgender status disclosure involving parents), 12 were specific to sports participation bans, and 9 were related to bathroom bans. The impact of such antitransgender policies extends far beyond legal and political spheres; it is a critical public health crisis that threatens not only access to care but also the physical and mental well-being and survival of the more than 1.6 million transgender people in the United States.[3]

At the core of this crisis is the deliberate denial of basic human rights and autonomy of a population for a malevolent, politically convenient, and irrational agenda. While the provision of gender affirmation (i.e., services that encompass a range of psychological, behavioral, medical, or legal interventions designed to support one's gender identity) remains highly politicized, we, as scientific, medical, and legal communities must learn to combat the spread of disinformation and misinformation on this topic as well as policies that purposefully mischaracterize the science. The current wealth of evidence, as supported by multiple established medical organizations like the American Medical Association and the current standards of transgender health care,[4] point to published findings indicating that high-quality, gender-affirming care is an integral protective factor for the mental health and well-being of transgender persons. This evidence also supports the view that gender-affirming care is part of bodily autonomy such that decisions are to be made only between transgender patients, providers, and parents of transgender youths—prioritizing parental consent and youths' assent.[4]

The impact of antitransgender legislation on the mental health of transgender individuals cannot be overstated. Transgender people face significant mental health challenges because of discrimination and stigma, and the banning of gender-affirming care, in particular, can lead to trauma and other severe mental health consequences, such as suicide attempts, severe psychological distress, and depression. These outcomes are six, eight, and nine times more prevalent, respectively, in transgender populations compared with the general population in the United States.[5,6] The denial of basic rights and freedoms only exacerbates these linkages, putting transgender communities at greater risk of mental health conditions.[6] In recent studies examining the impact of state policies, state-level antitransgender policies were significantly linked to more past-month psychological distress and endorsement of past-year suicidal thoughts, plans, and attempts among transgender adults—after adjusting for individual (e.g., demographics), interpersonal (e.g., experiences of transphobic discrimination), and social environmental (e.g., state-level inequality, religiosity as a proxy to social stigma) factors.[7] In another recent study, state-level and city-level protective policies were linked to significantly fewer experiences of discrimination.[8] These findings are concerning given their recency—that is, we are seeing these antitransgender policies drastically impacting mental health outcomes of transgender populations in the same year they are being introduced.

This is a crisis for public health and for mental health systems, in particular. Besides gender-affirming care itself, to our team's knowledge, there are currently no behavioral, social, or structural interventions tailored to transgender populations that have been demonstrated to prevent or reduce adverse mental health symptoms and outcomes.[6,9] To buffer the impact of antitransgender policies nationwide, greater resources must be invested in scalable interventions to improve family support, promote social connectedness, and build transgender individuals' and communities' capacity for empowerment and resistance.[10,11]

The physical and physiological health consequences of antitransgender legislation are equally devastating. For instance, the denial of gender-affirming care can trigger and lead to myriad adverse physical and physiological health outcomes and consequences, such as hormone imbalances, increased cancer risk, and increased risk of HIV and other sexually transmitted infections.[6] Indeed, some states have reported a chilling effect amid the enforcement of antitransgender policies, leaving providers and mental health professionals concerned that their practices might be penalized and that their patients' health and safety might be jeopardized.[12] Similar chilling effects have occurred in that transgender patients have hesitated to seek necessary care beyond gender-affirming care such as primary care or routine health checkups for fear of being targeted.[12] In addition, these antitransgender policies may force transgender persons who cannot flee to sanctuary states to conceal their transgender identities and disengage from lifesaving care, thus leading to unmitigated health-harming effects. These antitransgender policies can lead to increased rates of violence and victimization, too, which can result in physical injuries and trauma. As political motivations drive an antitransgender policy landscape, public sentiment follows, emboldening hate groups and dangerous subpopulations in society who wish to eradicate transgender people.

PUBLIC HEALTH ROLES AND EVIDENCE-BASED SOLUTIONS

We have at our disposal the ability and tools across scientific, medical, and legal armamentaria to proactively curb the impact of this legislation on the mental and physical health outcomes in transgender populations, and even dismantle the oppressive systems that uphold and reinforce these policies.[13] Strategic responses require us first to repair and heal relationships of historical distrust between transgender communities and scientific and medical communities. Forming meaningful collaborations and partnerships between transgender communities, stakeholders, and researchers entails establishing equitable team structures. These collaborative teams should prioritize transgender researchers and stakeholders as leaders in decision-making processes—while simultaneously being proactive in allyship, particularly those of us in leadership positions who are in power to amplify key and informed public health messages to make lasting changes.

Investing in community-engaged and community-led research, programs, and policy initiatives (e.g., the Trans Legislation Tracker, Center for Applied Trans Studies) is also crucial to ensure that such responses are community-driven and that they saliently address pressing health and legal needs and directly benefit transgender communities.[2,13] In addition, it is important to collaborate with other health equity scholars exploring and expanding concepts and strategies on resilience, racial equity, disability rights, Indigenous well-being, and reproductive health, among other topics, given the intertwining impacts of transgender health and policies in these areas,[13] and that health and legal professionals will also encounter transgender people among their target population.

Increased investments in rigorous research methodologies are necessary to strengthen evidence, address research and policy gaps, and combat misinformation. Specifically, these investments can begin with federal, state, and privately funded epidemiological studies or national surveys with gender-inclusive and gender-specific approaches that recognize and distinguish the health needs of all gender groups, longitudinal cohort studies that comprehensively map the impact of structural factors like protected policies on health, and interventions and clinical trials that are scalable and community-driven. These methodological and structural strategies can advance our responses and promote practices that are not only equitable but also just, on a larger scale.

Antitransgender policies reflect malicious attempts by those in power to pit the public against a highly marginalized group and avoid addressing critical economic and social issues that affect everyone (e.g., housing stability, infrastructure maintenance and expansion, climate change). The epidemic of antitransgender policies aims to regress decades of medical, public health, and policy progress, placing our achievements at a perilous crossroads. Where there is legislation that restricts a specific population's lives and human rights, there are multiple negative and inequitable consequences—as with the case of banning abortion rights, adverse birth outcomes and increased mortality were a consequence.[14] Respect for privacy, bodily autonomy, and the preservation of human rights for transgender people must be core ethical components of current and future health policies, and communities of medical, public health, and policy professionals must proactively oppose legislation that undermines public health responses. These actions are necessary components to achieving health equity for all. AJPH

CORRESPONDENCE

Correspondence should be sent to Arjee Javellana Restar, PhD, MPH, Departments of Epidemiology and Health Systems and Population Health, Box 351619, University of Washington School of Public Health, 3980 15th Ave NE, Seattle, WA 98105 (e-mail: restar@uw.edu). Reprints can be ordered at https://ajph.org by clicking the "Reprints" link.

PUBLICATION INFORMATION

Full Citation: Restar AJ, Layland EK, Davis B, Thompson H, Streed C. The public health crisis state of transgender health care and policy. *Am J Public Health*. 2024;114(2):161–163.

Acceptance Date: October 31, 2023.

DOI: https://doi.org/10.2105/AJPH.2023.307523

CONTRIBUTORS

All authors significantly contributed to drafting, editing, and reviewing the article. A. J. Restar originated the presented idea and worked with all authors to generate the framework, outline, and key messages of the article.

ACKNOWLEDGMENTS

A. J. Restar is supported by the Research Education Institute for Diverse Scholars Program at Yale University School of Public Health, and funded by the National Institute of Mental Health (R25MH087217) and amfAR, the Foundation of AIDS Research. C. Streed Jr reports salary support from the Boston University School of Medicine Department of Medicine Career Investment Award, American Heart Association career development grant (AHA 20CDA35320148), Doris Duke Charitable Foundation (grant 2022061), and National Heart, Lung, and Blood Institute career development grant (NHLBI 1K01HL151902-01A1). We would like to acknowledge insight to this piece from Elle Lett, PhD, MA, MBiostat.

Note. This article does not represent the official view of the sponsors.

CONFLICTS OF INTEREST

C. Streed Jr reports consulting fees from EverlyWell (2020–present), L'Oreal (2023–present), and The Texas Health Institute (2022–present) unrelated to the work presented in this article.

REFERENCES

1. Movement Advancement Project. Where we call home: LGBT people in rural America. April 2019. Arcus Foundation. Available at: https://www.arcusfoundation.org/wp-content/uploads/2019/05/lgbt-rural-report.pdf. Accessed November 14, 2023.
2. Trans Legislation Tracker. What anti-trans bills passed in 2023? 2023. Available at: https://translegislation.com/bills/2023/passed. Accessed October 2, 2023.
3. Herman JL, Flores AR, O'Neill KK. How many adults and youth identify as transgender in the United States? The Williams Institute. 2022. Available at: https://williamsinstitute.law.ucla.edu/publications/trans-adults-united-states. Accessed November 14, 2023.
4. Coleman E, Radix A, Bouman W, et al. Standards of care for the health of transgender and gender diverse people, version 8. *Int J Transgend Health* 2022;23(suppl 1):S1–S259. https://doi.org/10.1080/26895269.2022.2100644
5. James S, Herman J, Rankin S, Keisling M, Mottet L, Anafi Ma. The report of the 2015 US transgender survey. 2016. The National Center for Transgender Equality. Available at: https://transequality.org/sites/default/files/docs/usts/USTS-Full-Report-Dec17.pdf. Accessed November 14, 2023.
6. Scheim AI, Baker KE, Restar AJ, Sell RL. Health and health care among transgender adults in the United States. *Annu Rev Public Health*. 2022;43(1):503–523. https://doi.org/10.1146/annurev-publhealth-052620-100313
7. Price MA, Hollinsaid NL, McKetta S, Mellen EJ, Rakhilin M. Structural transphobia is associated with psychological distress and suicidality in a large national sample of transgender adults. *Soc Psychiatry Psychiatr Epidemiol*. 2023:1–10. https://doi.org/10.1007/s00127-023-02482-4
8. Truszczynski M, Truszczynski N, Estevez RI, Elliott AE. Does policy matter? The impact of state and city anti-discrimination policy on the discrimination experiences of trans and nonbinary people. *Sex Res Soc Policy*. 2022;19(4):1786–1794. https://doi.org/10.1007/s13178-022-00762-3
9. Layland EK, Carter JA, Perry NS, et al. A systematic review of stigma in sexual and gender minority health interventions. *Transl Behav Med*. 2020;10(5):1200–1210. https://doi.org/10.1093/tbm/ibz200
10. Ryan C, Russell ST, Huebner D, Diaz R, Sanchez J. Family acceptance in adolescence and the health of LGBT young adults. *J Child Adolesc Psychiatr Nurs*. 2010;23(4):205–213. https://doi.org/10.1111/j.1744-6171.2010.00246.x
11. Thompson HM, Feasley K, Ortiz R, Reyes K, Seanior A, Karnik NS. An implementation of a community-engaged, group-level mental health pilot for Black and Latina transgender women. *Health Promot Pract*. 2023; epub ahead of print May 12, 2023. https://doi.org/10.1177/15248399231172191
12. Gordon CM. Caught in the middle: the care of transgender youth in Texas. *Pediatrics*. 2022;149(6):e2022057475. https://doi.org/10.1542/peds.2022-057475
13. Thompson HM, Wang TM, Talan AJ, Baker KE, Restar AJ. First they came for us all: responding to anti-transgender structural violence with collective, community-engaged, and intersectional health equity research and advocacy. *Health Educ Behav*. 2023; epub ahead of print September 25, 2023. https://doi.org/10.1177/10901981231201146
14. Stevenson AJ. The pregnancy-related mortality impact of a total abortion ban in the United States: a research note on increased deaths due to remaining pregnant. *Demography*. 2021;58(6):2019–2028. https://doi.org/10.1215/00703370-9585908

The Languages of Public Health: Student Perspectives on Terms, Communities, and Language

Falah Nayif Rashoka, RN, MS, MPH, Jesus Vasquez, MS, MPH, Blair E. Williams, MPA, MBA, Tyler J. Fuller, MTS, MPH, Preeti Juturu, BA, and Damilola Oluwemimo, BSc

ABOUT THE AUTHORS

Falah Nayif Rashoka is with the University of Nebraska Medical Center, University of Nebraska-Lincoln. Jesus Vasquez is with New York Medical College, Valhalla, NY. Blair E. Williams is with the Johns Hopkins Bloomberg School of Public Health, Baltimore, MD. Tyler J. Fuller is with Boston University, Boston, MA. Preeti Juturu is with the Los Angeles Fielding School of Public Health, University of California, Los Angeles. Damilola Oluwemimo is with Western Illinois University Macomb Campus. All authors are also with the AJPH Student Think Tank.

See also The Languages of Public Health, pp. 166–192.

The delicate interplay between language and communication is of paramount importance in public health. This sector grapples with many challenges, from the containment of epidemics to the championing of mental health advocacy and the mobilization of communities for preventive care. A precise and deliberate dialogue is essential to address these issues effectively, as it can shape perceptions, foster understanding, and inspire action. The importance of linguistic nuances is well recognized by public health academics and practitioners.

The curated collection of written work to follow originated from the *AJPH* Student Think Tank's call for papers focusing on the languages of public health. The articles push beyond typical academic discourse; they integrate research with the authentic experiences of students and their communities. Covering a spectrum of storytelling, they underscore language's crucial role in shaping health trajectories and promoting the well-being of communities.

TECHNICAL TERMS AND THEORETICAL CONSTRUCTS

The articles in this section reflect the broader theme of public health communication and accessibility, even though they address different methods, contexts, and populations.

"The Power of Poetry: Rethinking How We Use Language in Global Health Research" by Woodson (p. 168) explores how applying poetic inquiry methodology can make scientific findings accessible and expressive, with examples from Peru's Marañón community, making it a tool for advancing social justice and decolonization. "When Public Health Terms Become Vernacular" by Matangi (p. 186) takes those ideas further by making public health terms relevant and relatable and showing that newly acquired "education creates opportunities for self-advocacy."

"Vulnerabilized: Revisiting the Language of the Vulnerable Populations Framework" by Garrett and Altman (p. 177) recounts how overly academic terms sometimes perpetuate narratives, influence attitudes, and alter priorities with disregard for systemic factors. Carter, in "The Resignation on Race" (p. 173), argues against oversimplifying correlations of health outcomes with racial groupings because this suggests that differences are innate rather than social consequences. In "Imagery as a Participatory Tool of Resilience for Marginalized Persons," Adan (p. 188) urges amplifying marginalized individuals' voices to achieve health equity.

Finally, "Public Health Preparedness Practitioners: Fluent in Disaster" (Kuddes; p. 180) underscores language fluency in disaster response, urging practitioners to comprehend and use diverse languages and understand their literal and metaphorical meanings so they can, ultimately, aid affected communities.

STUDENTS FROM MINORITIZED COMMUNITIES

Several articles explore the challenge that arises when individuals clearly understand the language they prefer but outsiders in the public health system may not, furthering the need for inclusive systems that consider these differences.

"Medical Etymology: A Journey of Identity" (Mitchell; p. 183) explores how terminology from "scholars of a bygone age" still influences specific health conditions and how communities can build solidarity and resources around a disability identity. "Public Health's Language Incompatibility With Veterans" by Henson (p. 175) delves deeper into the language gaps from erroneous beliefs about veterans and the misinterpretations that can occur when veterans use humor, jeopardizing their access to care and survival if the system cannot adapt. Harvey's "'We're Here, We're Queer, Get Used to It': Advancing LGBTQ+ Inclusive Language in Public Health" (p. 170) illustrates how reclaiming language can promote justice, remove stigma, and improve the quality of scientific research for LGBTQ+ (lesbian, gay, bisexual, transgender/-sexual, queer or questioning, and all subsects) individuals.

MULTILINGUAL STUDENTS

Finally, in the last theme of this year's articles, students reflect on health access when individuals and communities are constrained by limited English proficiency.

In "Unseen and Unheard: Increasing the Visibility of Limited English Proficiency Individuals Through a Language Justice Framework," Jilu (p. 190) highlights the importance of using a language justice framework in public health research, underscoring its role in meeting the needs of limited English-speaking proficiency communities. In "One Afternoon at a Vaccination Clinic," Muller (p. 184) recounts the significant challenges faced by individuals with limited English-speaking proficiency when they needed to communicate in a second language to access health care because a linguistically diverse workforce or resources were absent.

This collection of articles underscores the human aspect of language—how it can bridge gaps, foster understanding, and drive informed action. The overarching message remains clear: the language of public health serves as a tool for promoting inclusivity and positive change. AJPH

CORRESPONDENCE

Correspondence should be sent to Blair E. Williams, 12407 N MoPac Expy, Suite 250, PMB 375, Austin, TX 78758 (e-mail: bwill195@jhu.edu). Reprints can be ordered at http://www.ajph.org by clicking the "Reprints" link.

PUBLICATION INFORMATION

Full Citation: Rashoka FN, Vasquez J, Williams BE, Fuller TJ, Juturu P, Oluwemimo D. The languages of public health: student perspectives on terms, communities, and language. *Am J Public Health*. 2024;114(2):164–165.

Acceptance Date: November 20, 2023.

DOI: https://doi.org/10.2105/AJPH.2023.307545

CONTRIBUTORS

F.N. Rashoka, J. Vasquez, and B.E. Williams led the drafting of the editorial. T.J. Fuller and P. Juturu led the call for student perspectives and contributed critical content to the editorial. D. Oluwemimo contributed to the editorial. As members of the AJPH Student Think Tank, all authors contributed to the conceptualization of the Languages of Public Health theme and the selection of student submissions.

ACKNOWLEDGMENTS

We wish to thank Alfredo Morabia, editor in chief of *AJPH*, and the *AJPH* editorial staff for their support of the *AJPH* Student Think Tank.

CONFLICTS OF INTEREST

The authors have no conflicts of interest to disclose.

The Languages of Public Health: Avoiding a Modern-Day "Tower of Babel"

Robert J. Kim-Farley, MD, MPH

ABOUT THE AUTHOR

Robert J. Kim-Farley is an associate editor of AJPH *and is a professor-in-residence at the Fielding School of Public Health, University of California, Los Angeles.*

See also The Languages of Public Health, pp. 164–192.

AJPH February 2024, Vol. 114, No. 2

Language is the powerful tool that shapes our thoughts, perceptions, and interactions with the world and people. As noted in the *AJPH* Student Think Tank "Call for Papers," the words and languages we use can have a profound impact on how we understand public health theoretical constructs, populations, organizations, therapies, and diseases.

The story of the Tower of Babel (Figure 1) in Genesis 11:1–9 is a parable to explain why the people of the world speak different languages and highlights the power of language in shaping our understanding of the world. Language, therefore, is not just a tool for communication; it shapes our perceptions and interactions with the world around us and can also be a source of miscommunication when people are unable to understand each other.

In public health, language plays a critical role in shaping our thinking, collaboration, and interventions. The terms and acronyms we use inform our understanding. By being mindful of the language we use in public health discourse, both within the profession and with the individuals and communities we serve, we can promote greater understanding and collaboration among stakeholders. We can also be more sensitive and try to avoid situations where persons and groups are simply "talking over each other" and attempt to find common ground and nuances rather than polarizing language of "mandates" versus "individual freedoms."

Recent evidence suggests that even one's mother tongue can influence the way one thinks about many aspects of the world, including space and time[1]; this implies that language can influence how we perceive and categorize the world around us. Culture also shapes language and our worldviews, which can complicate efforts to translate some public health and other scientific concepts across languages. For example, the concept of "mental illness" may not exist in some cultures or may be stigmatized, making it more challenging for public health to address.[2]

In public health, the term "social determinants of health" is now a widely used concept in both research and practice to refer to the conditions in which we are born, grow, live, work, play, and age that affect health outcomes. Future research needs to further explore the role that language may play in identifying key factors contributing to health disparities and the ways in which public health should design and implement interventions to address them. Even artificial intelligence, especially large language models with natural language-processing features, may become increasingly useful to "identify vulnerable and at-risk populations . . . develop optimal recommendations/interventions . . . identify best practices . . . evaluate the benefits of health interventions . . . and to provide situational awareness."[3(p163)]

It is important to recognize that language can also be a source of misunderstanding and miscommunication in public health. For example, such terms as "obesity" or "overweight" can be stigmatizing for individuals who are affected by these conditions, and acronyms such as MSM (men who have sex with men) can be problematic because they do not fully capture the diversity of sexual identities and behaviors among this population. In 2022, the term "monkey pox" was changed by the World Health Organization to "mpox" because of concerns about "racist and stigmatizing language online."[4] It is important to develop and use language that is clear, accurate, nonstigmatizing, culturally appropriate, and inclusive.

In this special section of editorials submitted in response to the *AJPH* Student Think Tank, a variety of student authors demonstrate a wide diversity of perspectives, often from a lived experience, of how the languages of public health affect our professional and personal lives. Instead of dividing people by language, public health needs to bring people together by allowing them to understand each other despite their linguistic differences. We need to be mindful of the language we use in

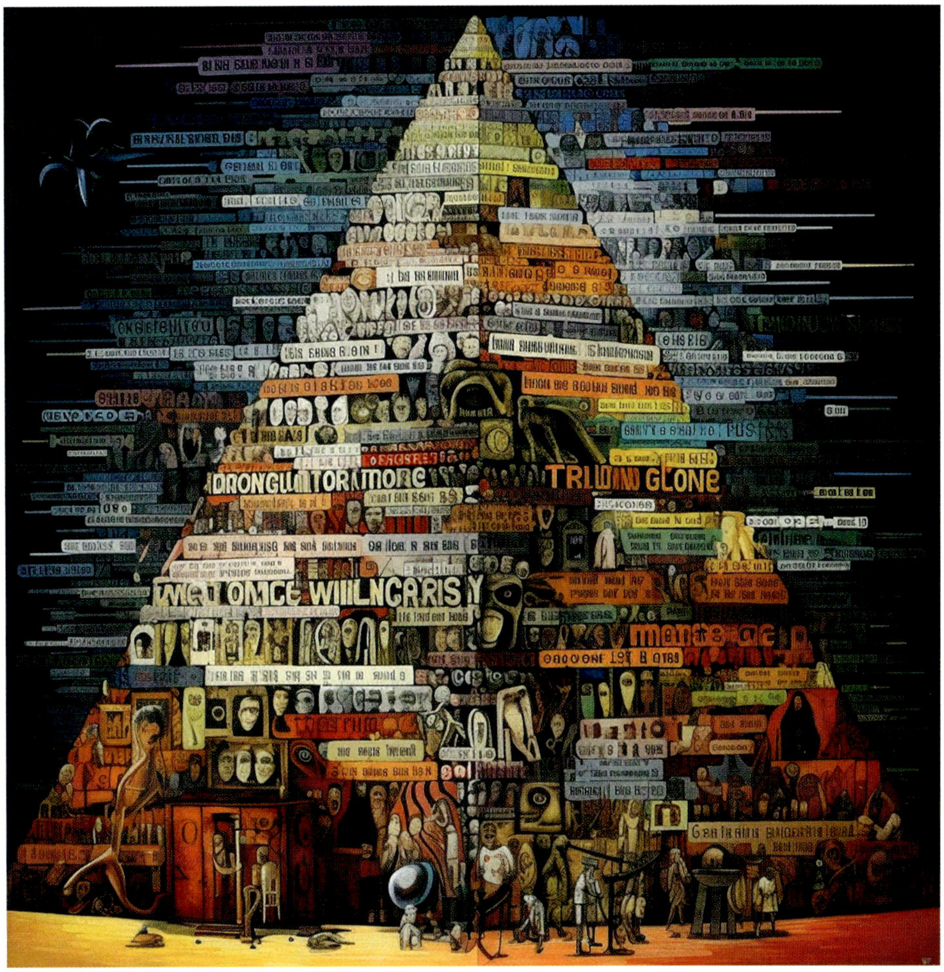

FIGURE 1— An Artificial Intelligence–Generated Image From a Text Prompt of a "Tower of Babel With Different Languages"

NOTE. This image is the first instance of using an AI-generated image in *AJPH*.

public health discourse to promote a greater understanding and collaboration—and not build a modern-day "Tower of Babel." AJPH

CORRESPONDENCE

Correspondence should be sent to Robert Kim-Farley, 4037 Rogen Dr, Encino, CA 91436 (e-mail: robert@kimfarley.org). Reprints can be ordered at http://www.ajph.org by clicking the "Reprints" link.

PUBLICATION INFORMATION

Full Citation: Kim-Farley RJ. The languages of public health: avoiding a modern-day "Tower of Babel". *Am J Public Health*. 2024;114(2): 166–167.

Acceptance Date: November 19, 2023.

DOI: https://doi.org/10.2105/AJPH.2023.307539

ACKNOWLEDGMENTS

I acknowledge the excellent work of the AJPH Student Think Tank members who worked so diligently in preparing this special section on the Languages of Public Health and for their helpful suggestions and comments on the original draft of this manuscript.

I acknowledge and disclose the use of Midjourney, an artificial intelligence (AI) text-to-image generating program, to create the "Tower of Babel" image with different languages, and the many eras of art and artists that served as a basis of AI learning.

CONFLICTS OF INTEREST

The author has no conflicts of interest to disclose.

REFERENCES

1. Boroditsky L. How language shapes thought. *Scientific American*. February 1, 2011. Available at: https://www.scientificamerican.com/article/how-language-shapes-thought. Accessed November 13, 2023.
2. Office of the Surgeon General, Center for Mental Health Services, National Institute of Mental Health. Mental health: culture, race, and ethnicity: a supplement to mental health: a report of the surgeon general. Chapter 2. Culture counts: the influence of culture and society on mental health. Substance Abuse and Mental Health Services Administration. August 2001. Available at: https://www.ncbi.nlm.nih.gov/books/NBK44249. Accessed November 13, 2023.
3. Baclic O, Tunis M, Young K, Doan C, Swerdfeger H, Schonfeld J. Challenges and opportunities for public health made possible by advances in natural language processing. *Can Commun Dis Rep*. 2020; 46(6):161–168. https://doi.org/10.14745/ccdr.v46i06a02
4. World Health Organization. WHO recommends new name for monkeypox disease. November 28, 2022. Available at: https://www.who.int/news/item/28-11-2022-who-recommends-new-name-for-monkeypox-disease. Accessed November 13, 2023.

The Power of Poetry: Rethinking How We Use Language in Global Health Research

Lisa Labita Woodson, MPH

ABOUT THE AUTHOR

Lisa Labita Woodson is a PhD epidemiology/global health candidate at the University of Arizona, Tucson.

See also The Languages of Public Health, pp. 164–192.

We use language to convey messages, concepts, and ideas. As researchers, we employ language in the scholarly pursuit of broadening our collective knowledge, usually in the form of scientific papers. However, this pathway of knowledge sharing is limited in its scope, outreach, and public accessibility. Consider the potential if we were to utilize language differently.

THE POWER OF POETRY

Recently, I was challenged to find ways to enhance the prominence of our research to foster greater engagement and connection to a more diverse audience. As a graduate student working in Peru's Amazon Basin, I wrestled with how to communicate the rich and nuanced experiences of my study participants while providing a platform to elevate their voices. This experience deepened my interest and investment in learning about different forms of art-based research, specifically poetry, as both a methodological approach and an advocacy tool for social change and decolonization.[1,2]

The poet Rita Dove once said, "Poetry is language at its most distilled and most powerful."[3] As researchers, how do we harness this power? This inquiry eventually led me to poetic inquiry, a form of research poetry that has been gaining traction over the past two decades and promoted by prominent researchers such as Prendergast, Bulter-Kisber, Van Rooyen, and Faulkner. It is a methodology that presents scientific findings in a more accessible and emotive format and helps to articulate the rich contextual realities of participants' lives through poetry.[4] It encourages greater introspection as researchers examine their research processes, their relationship to participants, and power dynamics.[5] Not only can it be used to draw attention to injustices and inequalities by articulating the lived experiences of those often marginalized and underrepresented,[6,7] but it is also an effective decolonization strategy within research that "delinks conformist methodologies of knowledge production and reconfigures the relations of power that shape conventional research by invigorating the (often suppressed) voice of the colonized."[2(p13)] For example, poetic inquiry has been used to deconstruct Western ideas of illness and disability in Palestine,[8] to explore transwomen identities in Namibia,[6] and as a tool to understanding how mobile money systems are perceived by users in rural Kenya.[9]

Currently, several scientific journals publish poetry including the *JAMA Poetry and Medicine* and *Health Promotion Practice*. Poetry was also used to promote COVID-19 vaccination through the *Dear Vaccine* project (https://www.globalvaccinepoem.com). Recently, St Louis University jointly with Texas A&M University launched a biannual poetry journal in public health called *Leaders Igniting Generational Healing and Transformation* or LIGHT (https://light4ph.org). This highlights the growing public and academic interest in the intersection of poetry and public health. However, to the best of my knowledge, there is no centralized global health repository of poetry that is publicly available. Through a preliminary, and by no means rigorous, search, only a handful of articles and publications appeared across search engines and databases with the keywords of "global health" and "anthology" or "poetry" or "poems" or "poetic inquiry."

Yet, poetic inquiry does not come without thoughtful reflection on the methodological boundaries and quality of this language form. Specifically, we must consider if we are creating good poetry and, correspondingly, if the data are still trustworthy, persuasive, and credible.[10] This remains a highly debated topic among research poets and poet researchers alike. Despite being new to this field, I see inherent value in poetry. It is exactly what is needed right now in the field of global health, and more expansively in public health research. It positions us as researchers within the research, provides a space for reflexivity, and helps humanize the experience of our participants. In addition, it compels us to consider the oft-neglected local and cultural contexts of our research and to question dominant Eurocentric narratives.[11] Using this form of compact and emotive language has the potential to make us better researchers.

INTERSECTION OF POETRY AND RESEARCH

To conclude, here is an original poem I wrote following a field visit to study sites in Loreto, Peru, along the Marañón River, a major tributary of the Amazon River. My research focused on the downstream impacts of COVID-19 mitigation efforts on adolescent pregnancy in one of the country's impoverished regions marked by a high rate of adolescent pregnancy and poor maternal and child health indicators.[12] It outlined pathways that connect the risk of adolescent pregnancy to several ecological system factors from the macro, micro, and individual levels such as poverty, lack of education and health care access, and social and gender norms that limited female autonomy and helped to conserve the practice of early unions. In addition, communities faced new challenges posed by the widespread adoption of technology among adolescents amplified during the pandemic. This poem weaves together different lived experiences of young girls in the Amazon synthesized from data collected from interviews and focus group discussions with adolescents, *apus* or community leaders, and educators, as well as secondary data sources and field observations.

Marañón

Heavy rain floods through open windows
puddles across the wooden plank floor
traffic worn from chickens and children
impatient for the season's end
as they wait like islands on the Marañón.

A pregnant girl rests her swollen body
across the warped metal rocker
careful to balance her weight while
pushing her feet firmly onto the ground
and her back to the chair's spine.

In the dry season, she had played
voley in the open fields before her
that now pool above her waist
threatening to swallow the bodies of girls
too young to carry to term.

In the secret pleasures of the *oscura*,
he had exposed her with his body's weight
and used his cell phone to examine her
pubescent breasts before abandoning her
for *otro trabajo* down the Marañón.

Yet she still waits, days swollen by tears
she does not cry but floods the haul
of the *peke peke* used to carry her body
upriver to Nauta's eroded oil-slicked banks
but not time enough to save her
—and her unborn child.

AJPH

CORRESPONDENCE

Correspondence should be sent to Lisa Labita Woodson, 1295 N Martin Ave, Tucson, AZ 85724 (e-mail: lisalabita@arizona.edu). Reprints can be ordered at https://ajph.org by clicking the "Reprints" link.

PUBLICATION INFORMATION

Full Citation: Woodson LL. The power of poetry: rethinking how we use language in global health research. *Am J Public Health*. 2024;114(2): 168–169.

Acceptance Date: October 7, 2023.

DOI: https://doi.org/10.2105/AJPH.2023.307495

ACKNOWLEDGMENTS

Research in the Peruvian Amazon was supported and funded by the Fulbright-Fogarty and Global Health Equity Scholar fellowships (grant D43TW010540).

I would like to thank the community health workers of Universidad Peruana Cayetano Heredia's project *Mamás del Río*, *apus* or community leaders, local health staff, teachers, and adolescents in my study sites for their contributions to my research and, in turn, the inspiration for this poem. A special thanks to my research assistant, Adriana Garcia Saldivar; my *Beyond Global Health* co-collaborators, Shameka Poetry Thomas and Purnima Madhivanan; and mentors, Magaly Blas, Priscilla Magrath, and Heidi Brown.

CONFLICTS OF INTEREST

The author declared no conflicts of interest.

REFERENCES

1. Faulkner SL. Poetic inquiry. In: Leavy P, ed. *Handbook of Arts-Based Research.* New York, NY: Guilford Publications; 2017:208–230.
2. Van Rooyen H, D'Abdon R. Transforming data into poems: poetic inquiry practices for social and human sciences. *Education as Change.* 2020;24:1–17. https://doi.org/10.25159/1947-9417/8103
3. Streitfeld D. Laureate for a new age. *Washington Post.* May 19, 1993;19.
4. Richardson L. Poetic representation of interviews. In: Gubrium JF, Holstein JA, eds. *Postmodern Interviewing.* Thousand Oaks, CA: SAGE; 2003:187–201.
5. Fernández-Giménez ME, Jennings LB, Wilmer H. Poetic inquiry as a research and engagement method in natural resource science. *Society Nat Resour.* 2019;32(10):1080–1091. https://doi.org/10.1080/08941920.2018.1486493
6. van Rooyen H, Essack Z, Mahali A, Groenewald C, Solomons A. "The power of the poem": using poetic inquiry to explore trans-identities in Namibia. *Arts Health.* 2021;13(3):315–328. https://doi.org/10.1080/17533015.2020.1805634
7. Petteway RJ, Burch SR, Dill LJ. Altering auras, ideas, and dreams: naming and (re)claiming a poetry for the public's health. *Health Promot Pract.* 2022;23(4):537–542. https://doi.org/10.1177/15248399221105793
8. Alshammari S. Disability as metaphor or resilience: a Palestinian poetic inquiry. *J Int Intercult Commun.* 2022;15(4):362–373. https://doi.org/10.1080/17513057.2022.2114528
9. McBride N, Liyala S. Memoirs from Bukhalalire: a poetic inquiry into the lived experience of M-PESA mobile money usage in rural Kenya. *Eur J Inf Syst.* 2023;32(2):173–194. https://doi.org/10.1080/0960085X.2021.1924088
10. Faulkner SL. *Poetic Inquiry: Craft, Method and Practice.* New York, NY: Routledge; 2019.
11. Aubel J, Chibanda D. The neglect of culture in global health research and practice. *BMJ Glob Health.* 2022;7(9):e009914. https://doi.org/10.1136/bmjgh-2022-009914
12. Instituto Nacional de Estadística e Informática. *Encuesta Demografica y de Salud Familiar - ENDES 2019.* 2019. Available at: https://www.inei.gob.pe/media/MenuRecursivo/publicaciones_digitales/Est/Endes2019. Accessed October 27, 2023.

"We're Here, We're Queer, Get Used to It": Advancing LGBTQ+-Inclusive Language in Public Health

Tyler D. Harvey, MPH

ABOUT THE AUTHOR

Tyler D. Harvey is with the Yale School of Medicine, New Haven, CT.

See also The Languages of Public Health, pp. 164–192.

I recently had my annual physical with a new doctor—an experience any queer or transgender person knows to be anxiety-provoking. Before going into it, I asked myself: How much do I share? Should I be honest about certain things, or should I do what needs to be done to get out as quickly as possible? I decided to go with the former this time, writing down "queer" when asked my gender on the intake form. Minutes later, I found myself responding to questions from the doctor about my gender identity—all of which had nothing to do with my visit that day. Leaving, I felt regret, frustrated at the doctor and myself. This experience reminded me that the language used in clinical and public health settings remains limited for me as an individual from the lesbian, gay, bisexual, transgender, and queer (LGBTQ+) community.

This was not my first negative experience with a doctor and probably will not be my last. Unfortunately, these experiences are not unique to me. It has been shown that the health system is particularly ill-equipped to deal with the unique needs of LGBTQ+ individuals.[1] A survey of US academic medical institutions found that only 16% reported having comprehensive LGBTQ+-competency training within their faculty practices.[2] Given this, LGBTQ+ people often find navigating the health system difficult, and discrimination within health care spaces negatively influences the health-seeking behaviors of LGBTQ+ people.[3] In a nationally representative sample of 1828 LGBTQ+ people, one in five reported delaying medical care because of discrimination within the health system.[4] There are many needed reforms to improve LGBTQ+ health, and one of those centers on the words we allow people to use to describe themselves.

Despite recent increased sociocultural acceptance surrounding LGBTQ+ issues and a greater percentage of Americans identifying as LGBTQ+, the field of public health as a whole still lags behind in adapting and implementing appropriate, inclusive language for the whole range of LGBTQ+ identities.[5] Some systems, particularly ones focused on LGBTQ+ health, such as Fenway Health in Boston, are leading the ways in such efforts.[6] But, for the most part, public health surveys, national studies, and medical forms overlook us, either not including any questions regarding diverse sexual and gender identity at all or including ones that are flawed.

Here, I present two arguments regarding the implications around the lack of LGBTQ+-inclusive language in public health: (1) it is an injustice, and (2) it is bad for science.

INJUSTICE

Increasingly, LGBTQ+ individuals are using nontraditional labels for their sexual and gender identities. These include labels such as queer, pansexual, and genderfluid. Survey data of 17 000 LGBTQ+ youths found that more than one in four identified with such nontraditional labels.[7] But these terms have not always been embraced by our community, and some may still find them offensive. For example, the first documented use of the word "queer" was in 1895 when writer Oscar Wilde was on trial for homosexual acts.[8] During the trial, a letter from the Marquis of Queensberry was read describing his disgust for homosexuality—including Wilde's relationship with his own son—by calling them "Snob Queers." The term was then widely adapted as a derogatory term in the media.[8] Using language—in this case and many others—was a mechanism to exert control and enact shame.

In recent years, though, we—as a community—have moved to reclaim terms that have been used against us. For example, the term "queer" was reclaimed by activists and organizations such as Queer Nation during the AIDS epidemic in the 1980s and '90 s. Reclaiming it was meant to be a process of intensity, expressing anger at the discrimination LGBTQ+ communities were faced with during the AIDS crisis.[9]

Today, many in the LGBTQ+ community view queer as an inclusive, umbrella term—rather than an exclusionary one—that captures various identities.[9] Queer is one example of the ever-evolving nature of language surrounding the LGBTQ+ community.

Thus, the manners in which public health allow LGBTQ+ individuals to identify themselves is intrinsically one of power, and it is an injustice if appropriate labels are not presented for LGBTQ+ people. Self-determination in how people are addressed has long been linked to a history of oppression. To be able to determine how one labels oneself is to exert authority over them. If the language of public health does not even present options that appropriately and fully include us, how can we ever be truly represented? It is a moral failure of the field.

BAD FOR SCIENCE

To my second point, not appropriately capturing sexual and gender identity produces inaccurate scientific findings. For example, surveys capturing sexual minority identity typically only use three options: "heterosexual," "gay/lesbian," and "bisexual." What this means is that LGBTQ+ individuals identifying with neither gay/lesbian nor bisexual, are forced to select a category that is not only inaccurate but also increases the heterogeneity of subgroups within the LGBTQ+ community. This results in a misclassification error and biases LGBTQ+ health research.[10]

National data confirm this. West and McCabe found that associations between sexual identity and substance use behaviors were weakened when only three options ("heterosexual," "gay/lesbian," and "bisexual") were presented to survey respondents, as opposed to including a fourth option of "something else."[11] Qualitative data reinforce that current data collection tools are too limited in scope.[12] The quantitative erasure of LGBTQ+ people from health studies—ones that are typically funded with our taxpayer dollars—is not only harmful toward the LGBTQ+ community but also requires us to interpret the whole body of evidence surrounding LGBTQ+ health based on how sexual and gender identity was captured in those studies.

MOVING FORWARD

I have several recommendations for public health professionals and researchers to update our language to be more inclusive for LGBTQ+ individuals. First, all federally funded data-collection tools should be required to appropriately collect data on sexual and gender minority identities, just as any other demographic variable like age, race/ethnicity, and education level. Second, data collection tools should include diverse, exhaustive response options. This would mean providing an open-response option allowing people to write in their identity rather than only selecting predetermined categories. Last, as identity is fluid, it is important to test the validity of various response options and continue to monitor their performance over time.

Broad adaptation of LGBTQ+-inclusive language in public health will require effort, intentionality, and costs. Among many things, it will require medical and public health practitioners to educate themselves on the diversity of the LGBTQ+ community and understand how this diversity shapes their work. It requires updating public health data collection tools—from federally funded surveys to government intake forms. New survey tools will require time and resources invested from funding agencies, such as the National Institutes of Health, to be empirically sound. Relatedly, LGBTQ+ community members must also have an important role in this work by serving on health care advisory panels, data equity workgroups, and community-led groups to help inform the use of such inclusive language. All of these activities and more must be done to advance the field toward justice and generate quality science.

For many LGBTQ+ people, including myself, the language we choose to describe who we are is deeply personal. For me, queer represents my sexual and gender identity but also a political identity rooted in demands for equality and liberation for our community. As legislation across the United States attacks LGBTQ+ rights, I find it more important now than ever to be able to correctly identify myself. I will use the same words queer and transgender people did 50 years ago as their friends, lovers, and chosen family died during the AIDS crisis because of a failed government response: "We're here, we're queer, get used to it." We all have an obligation to push public health toward more inclusive language for LGBTQ+ individuals if we want to make any progress in advancing health equity and producing high-quality science. AJPH

CORRESPONDENCE

Correspondence should be sent to Tyler D. Harvey, MPH, 333 Cedar St, New Haven, CT, 06511 (e-mail: tyler.harvey@yale.edu). Reprints can be ordered at https://ajph.org by clicking the "Reprints" link.

PUBLICATION INFORMATION

Full Citation: Harvey TD. "We're here, we're queer, get used to it": advancing LGBTQ+-inclusive language in public health. *Am J Public Health*. 2024; 114(2):170–172.

Acceptance Date: November 15, 2023.

DOI: https://doi.org/10.2105/AJPH.2023.307529

ACKNOWLEDGMENTS

The author would like to acknowledge the OpEd-Project in partnership with AcademyHealth for their support through the Public Voices fellowship during the writing of this editorial.

They would like to also thank Randi Hutter Epstein, MD, MPH, writer in residence at the Yale School of Medicine, for guidance on the final version of this piece.

CONFLICTS OF INTEREST

The author has no conflicts of interest to disclose.

REFERENCES

1. Pratt-Chapman ML, Eckstrand K, Robinson A, et al. Developing standards for cultural competency training for health care providers to care for lesbian, gay, bisexual, transgender, queer, intersex, and asexual persons: consensus recommendations from a national panel. *LGBT Health*. 2022;9(5):340–347. https://doi.org/10.1089/lgbt.2021.0464
2. Khalili J, Leung LB, Diamant AL. Finding the perfect doctor: identifying lesbian, gay, bisexual, and transgender–competent physicians. *Am J Public Health*. 2015;105(6):1114–1119. https://doi.org/10.2105/AJPH.2014.302448
3. Carpenter E. "The health system just wasn't built for us": queer cisgender women and gender expansive individuals' strategies for navigating reproductive health care. *Womens Health Issues*. 2021;31(5):478–484. https://doi.org/10.1016/j.whi.2021.06.004
4. Medina C, Mahowald L. *Discrimination and Barriers to Well-Being: The State of the LGBTQI+ Community in 2022*. Washington, DC: Center for American Progress; 2022.
5. Jones JM. LGBT identification rises to 5.6% in latest US estimate. *Gallup News*. 2021:24.
6. Bradford J, Cahill S, Grasso C, Makadon H. How to gather data on sexual orientation and gender identity in clinical settings. Boston, MA: The Fenway Institute; 2012.
7. Watson RJ, Wheldon CW, Puhl RM. Evidence of diverse identities in a large national sample of sexual and gender minority adolescents. *J Res Adolesc*. 2020;30(suppl 2):431–442. https://doi.org/10.1111/jora.12488
8. Clarke M. *'Queer' History: A History of Queer*. College Park, MD: The National Archives; 2021.
9. Perlman M. How the word "queer" was adopted by the LGBTQ community. *Columbia Journalism Review*. January 22, 2019. https://www.cjr.org/language_corner/queer.php. Accessed January 3, 2024.
10. Lorenz TK. Relying on an "other" category leads to significant misclassification of sexual minority participants. *LGBT Health*. 2021;8(5):372–377. https://doi.org/10.1089/lgbt.2020.0449
11. West BT, McCabe SE. Choices matter: how response options for survey questions about sexual identity affect population estimates of its association with alcohol, tobacco, and other drug use. *Field Methods*. 2021;33(4):335–354. https://doi.org/10.1177/1525822X21998516
12. Bauer GR, Hammond R, Travers R, Kaay M, Hohenadel KM, Boyce M. "I don't think this is theoretical; this is our lives": how erasure impacts health care for transgender people. *J Assoc Nurses AIDS Care: JANAC*. 2009;20(5):348–361. https://doi.org/10.1016/j.jana.2009.07.004

The Resignation on Race

Christopher A. Carter, BS

ABOUT THE AUTHOR

Christopher A. Carter is with the Master of Public Health Program, Kansas State University, Manhattan.

See also The Languages of Public Health, pp. 164–192.

Public health has a racism problem—one that is neither new nor unique but that is encompassing and inhibitory. Correcting many aspects of racism requires large, systematic changes in policy built on sound evidence, but we have already made an error. Epidemiologists and other public health practitioners, in the effort to meaningfully categorize people to better understand why health outcomes differ between groups, often rely on racial classifications. In doing this, we concede a critical point: we accept the premise that race is a real, concrete, and unavoidable reality. We effectively resign, or "give in," to the harmful framework.

Race is a construct born of European colonialism and based on geographical, cultural, and religious attitudes rather than biology.[1] Contemporary Europeans encoded this construct into a new social contract, transforming race, as described by Berger and Luckmann in *The Social Construction of Reality*, from the subjective to the objective, from an idea to a social reality.[1,2] Despite this societal institutionalization, race remains an unscientific and erroneous classification system.[3]

Although constructed from subjectivity, this reality inflicts objective damage.[4] When we measure and report that damage using racial groupings, we give the appearance that these differences are innate and not a social, economic, or environmental consequence. We know that because people of color experience racism, are unheard, and are treated differently than White people they experience disparate health outcomes.[5] But that is not what we say. Instead, we compact all that nuance into a simple catchall. We simply say it is because of their race.

Some authors may report racial classifications as a proxy for other factors associated with race in the United States (e.g., socioeconomic status) or because those factors act as (unmeasured) confounders on study groups. However, these methods are problematic. First—more broadly—by using disproven racial classifications, we buy into a harmful framework and lend scientific credence to an unscientific system. This is antithetical to our goals of health equity and erodes trust in the communities we serve. Second, this framing passes the blame from systemic issues to "innate" differences, from change to resignation, an excuse. If the first step of fixing a problem is recognizing it, we are doing ourselves a disservice by failing to report the true cause of disparate health outcomes: racism, not race.

So how can we avoid errors regarding race? Synthesizing from Deadric T. William's 2019 commentary, scholars should properly contextualize race as a historical and social consequence; public health practitioners and policymakers should seek to better understand how racial concepts enforce Mill's racial contract; and researchers should, if using race-based grouping, investigate within-group variations.[6] These actions will combat the amplification of racial frameworks while also improving our understanding of health inequities. Ultimately, however, we must recognize the influence of systemic racism in public health and work to dismantle it.

Twenty-five years ago, in a commentary published in *AJPH*, Mindy Fullilove asked, "Why continue to accept something that is not only without biological merit but also full of evil social impact?"[7(p1297)] Addressing racism in public health requires, from all of us, reflection on our biases and action in rectifying our errors. This is the responsibility of leaders and policymakers, of editors and journalists, and of students and professors. By contextualizing race as a social construct, understanding its institutionalization, and accurately investigating and reporting its impacts, we can begin to rectify that evil. AJPH

CORRESPONDENCE

Correspondence should be sent to Christopher A. Carter, 103B Trotter Hall, 1710 Denison Ave, Manhattan, KS 66506 (e-mail: ccarter0@k-state.edu). Reprints can be ordered at http://www.ajph.org by clicking the "Reprints" link.

PUBLICATION INFORMATION

Full Citation: Carter CA. The resignation on race. *Am J Public Health*. 2024;114(2):173–174.

Acceptance Date: November 15, 2023.

DOI: https://doi.org/10.2105/AJPH.2023.307530

ACKNOWLEDGMENTS

The author thanks Justin Kastner for his continued and invaluable support and advice.

CONFLICTS OF INTEREST

The author reports no conflicts of interest.

REFERENCES

1. Mills CW. *The Racial Contract.* Ithaca, NY: Cornell University Press; 1997.
2. Berger PL, Luckmann T. *The Social Construction of Reality: A Treatise in the Sociology of Knowledge.* Garden City, NY: Anchor Books; 1966.
3. Kaufman JS, Cooper RS. Race in epidemiology: new tools, old problems. *Ann Epidemiol.* 2008; 18(2):119–123. https://doi.org/10.1016/j.annepidem.2007.09.002
4. Williams DR, Mohammed SA. Racism and health I: pathways and scientific evidence. *Am Behav Sci.* 2013;57(8):1152–1173. https://doi.org/10.1177/0002764213487340
5. Hoberman JM. *Black and Blue: The Origins and Consequences of Medical Racism.* Berkeley: University of California Press; 2012.
6. Williams DT. A call to focus on racial domination and oppression: a response to "Racial and Ethnic Inequality in Poverty and Affluence, 1959–2015." *Popul Res Policy Rev.* 2019;38(5): 655–663. https://doi.org/10.1007/s11113-019-09538-x
7. Fullilove MT. Comment: abandoning "race" as a variable in public health research—an idea whose time has come. *Am J Public Health.* 1998;88(9):1297–1298. https://doi.org/10.2105/AJPH.88.9.1297

Public Health's Language Incompatibility With Veterans

Taylor Henson, BS

ABOUT THE AUTHOR

Taylor Henson is with the Mel and Enid Zuckerman College of Public Health, University of Arizona, Tucson.

See also The Languages of Public Health, pp. 164–192.

I hear the calls, "Gas! Gas! Gas!" and sigh then drop into my defensive position to strap my gas mask on my face before haphazardly firing blanks into the Hawaiian jungle to simulate suppressing an attack. As a timid 19-year-old U.S. Marine, I struggled desperately in my marine squad leader course but ultimately made it through. My experiences as a rifleman are far from unique and are very tame compared with many. Despite this, upon separation, I could not help but feel like every journal I read about my community did not fully understand how to accurately capture the experience I had as a Marine. The journal articles felt like a form of attack, a written way to demean and belittle the people I most identified with. There is a language disconnect between the great minds of public health academia and the ever-present veteran issues that may inadvertently drive veterans further away from the initiatives designed to help them.

When discussing veteran public health concerns, it is impossible not to latch on to the topic of mental health in my community. There has been a rise in programs and research aimed at helping veterans suffering from the traumas of their service, and yet the suicide rate among veterans is 32 per 100 000, compared with 17.2 per 100 000 for nonveterans.[1] Inadvertently or not, the blame for these suicides is often placed on the veterans themselves through the language used in public health communications. For example, several articles discuss how veterans do not seek help because of their need to "be tough" or to "mask their feelings."[2] This blame can be traced back to stigma, a topic the public health community frequently attempts to combat. Although articles such as these are aimed at addressing the stigma veterans face, they can just as easily come across as using stigmatizing language. I have an abundance of memories of deep, heartfelt conversations with the Marines in Golf Company who were little more than acquaintances. The idea that veterans take on this robotic need to hide all emotion is based more on misunderstanding and fantastical media depictions of service members than it is on reality. Veterans are a community of communities, a collective of individuals from the most diverse of backgrounds. If approached with language they relate to, veterans can be helped like anyone else.

An excellent example of this would be the use of humor to approach heavier topics and convey information to the veteran community. The use of humor is a common coping mechanism veterans use to navigate difficult times. Understanding gallows humor, in particular, helps explain the disconnect between veterans' language usage and that of public health professionals. Gallows humor can best be described as humor that pokes fun at death or horrifying situations, and I cannot think of a better way to describe the humor used in the Marine Corps. The nonchalance about death and various other horrible situations is commonplace in much of the service. The threat of the public health community misunderstanding this mechanism of dealing with trauma is ever present in all veterans I know. Rather than assuming this is a morbid preoccupation, public health officials must begin to hear what veterans are saying—this is the only way many of us can cope with this overwhelming burden.[3] This issue stems from well-meaning public health professionals hearing dark, pessimistic-sounding language they are not familiar with and misidentifying it as suicidal ideation. It is important for the public health community at large to understand that this talk is not always a cause for immediate involuntary commitment or mental health holds; rather it is the only way some know how to cope.[3]

While working in public health, I often hear terms such as "resilience" being used to determine the susceptibility to suicide among veterans.[4] Although it is a near certainty that public health professionals participating in this research mean no harm by their use of "resilience," it is easy for a veteran to take offense to its usage. Its use suggests that veterans who died by suicide were simply less resilient than those who continue to live—a suggestion that could easily drive veterans away from public health initiatives. By contrast, when many veterans, including me,

AJPH February 2024, Vol. 114, No. 2

think of resilience, we do not think of succumbing to the weight of our trauma. I think of my time hiking for miles despite a crippling lack of electrolytes or making my squad members laugh after days of rain and wet gear with no end in sight. I am able to use the objectivity I have learned throughout my public health studies to understand what researchers mean by resilience, but from the perspective of a veteran, I can absolutely see where the language may lead to adverse outcomes.

Laying the information on the table, it is fair to say that this language gap leaves veterans to ponder how much veteran culture is taken into consideration and the efficacy of current public health interventions. It has been reported that of veterans who died by suicide in 2018, 63% did not utilize Veterans Affairs health care services even once for at least two years before their deaths.[1] Additionally, veterans are overrepresented in the unhoused population.[5] The Veterans Affairs touts its public health efforts when it cites the reduction in unhoused rates among veterans in recent years. Although true, this ignores that between 2017 and 2020 nearly 25% of veterans utilizing Veterans Affairs assisted housing programs were kicked out of the program because they suffered from a substance use disorder.[5] Ironically, there exists one set of statistics showing how the lack of services may correlate with the higher suicide rate and another set showing how the programs designed to help veterans remove veterans experiencing hardship with substance misuse. This conflicting language makes navigating veteran issues a struggle for someone pursuing a public health education, let alone those trying to understand the problems from the outside.

Some individuals may argue that nothing can be done to address this language disconnect between the public health community and veterans. However, veteran-targeted programs have room for improvement, and this work must be done by those who speak veterans' language. Like any public health intervention, community involvement must be the backbone. I would love to say that the best way to approach this disconnect would be to place veterans in areas of public health designed to address their personal issues, but that would be a Band-Aid, a short-term fix that does not teach public health officials how to navigate unfamiliar communities. The language gap is an area that can be filled, but to do so requires collaboration and mutual understanding between public health officials and the veteran community. In a world where common language in veteran populations may be seen as dark or unprofessional, it is hard for veterans to convey their individual issues in a manner that the public health community at large will respect. Until we as public health professionals take the initiative to understand the language used outside of academia, the veterans we aim to serve will continue to feel like foreign specimens for study, rather than people who have capably and honorably served our country and now need help. AJPH

CORRESPONDENCE

Correspondence should be sent to Taylor Henson, 1251 W. Calle De Cobre, Sahuarita, AZ 85629 (e-mail: hensontaylor13@gmail.com). Reprints can be ordered at http://www.ajph.org by clicking the "Reprints" link.

PUBLICATION INFORMATION

Full Citation: Henson T. Public health's language incompatibility with veterans. *Am J Public Health*. 2024;114(2):175–176.

Acceptance Date: November 15, 2023.

DOI: https://doi.org/10.2105/AJPH.2023.307531

CONFLICTS OF INTEREST

The author has no conflicts of interest to declare.

REFERENCES

1. Ramchand R. Suicide among veterans: veterans' issues in focus. *Rand Health Q*. 2022;9(3):21.
2. Kulesza M, Pedersen ER, Corrigan PW, Marshall GN. Help-seeking stigma and mental health treatment seeking among young adult veterans. *Mil Behav Health*. 2015;3(4):230–239. https://doi.org/10.1080/21635781.2015.1055866
3. Burek G. Military culture: working with veterans. *Am J Psychiatry*. 2018;13(9):3–5. https://doi.org/10.1176/appi.ajp-rj.2018.130902
4. Dorsey Holliman BA, Monteith LL, Spitzer EG, Brenner LA. Resilience, cultural beliefs, and practices that mitigate suicide risk among African American women veterans. *SAGE Open*. 2018;8(1). Available at: https://journals.sagepub.com/doi/epub/10.1177/2158244017753506. Accessed December 9, 2023. https://doi.org/10.1177/2158244017753506
5. Ellison ML, Schutt RK, Yuan L-H, et al. Impact of peer specialist services on residential stability and behavioral health status among formerly homeless veterans with cooccurring mental health and substance use conditions. *Med Care*. 2020;58(4):307–313. https://doi.org/10.1097/MLR.0000000000001284

Vulnerabilized: Revisiting the Language of the Vulnerable Populations Framework

Camryn M. Garrett, MPH, and Rochelle Altman, EdD

ABOUT THE AUTHORS

Both authors are with the Department of Health Promotion, Education, and Behavior, Arnold School of Public Health, University of South Carolina, Columbia. Camryn M. Garrett is also with the Center for Healthcare Quality, University of South Carolina, Columbia.

See also The Languages of Public Health, pp. 164–192.

Public health prioritizes the identification, mitigation, and elimination of health disparities, which are defined as preventable, inequitable differences in health risks and outcomes burdening socially disadvantaged populations. These patterns of disparities become more evident when aggregated from the individual to the population level. For example, Black women disproportionately face increased maternal morbidity and mortality outcomes as a result of social determinants of health, such as structural racism, social prejudices, biases, and policies.[1] Despite the urgent and ongoing need to address the underlying causes of these disparities, there remains a lack of formalized nomenclature that adequately encapsulates the complex, multifaceted systems that perpetuate vulnerability.[2] In response, we propose a novel technical term to augment the language of vulnerability.

Language that articulates differential risks among populations is rooted in the *Belmont Report*. This seminal document established protections to guard against the exploitation of vulnerable groups, specifically identifying "racial minorities, the economically disadvantaged, the very sick, and the institutionalized."[3] Building on the *Belmont Report*, the vulnerable populations framework situated individuals in the broader contexts of their communities and environments, recognizing the reciprocal relationships between the social determinants of health and health outcomes.[4] Although existing definitions define *vulnerability* as susceptibility to harm or resulting from external influence, its ubiquitous use has eroded its meaning, often overemphasizing the influence of individual attributes while diluting the deterministic role of upstream determinants.[5,6]

Although strides have been made to refine the concept of *vulnerability*, there remain challenges (e.g., inconsistency, ambiguity) and implications (e.g., gaps between theoretical and operational levels) that are necessary to consider when using vulnerability language and frameworks.[7] The language of vulnerability can be deleterious when placing undue, deficit-oriented emphasis at the individual level, as doing so conceals the role of systemic factors in creating the processes and environments through which individuals, who aggregate into populations, are made vulnerable.[8] Merely designating populations as vulnerable fails to identify the actions of systems of oppression that cause and maintain health disparities.

Recognizing this gap, we advocate a linguistic evolution from the passive adjective of *vulnerable* to the updated, transitive verb *vulnerabilize* to illustrate the ongoing process through which vulnerability is created and sustained. We define the term *vulnerabilized* as the outcomes of the processes, driven by distal systemic factors beyond the control of the individual or population, where heightened risks intersect and compound among various social identities and positions and result in differential, unjust, and preventable health differences.

Kimberlé Crenshaw coined the term *intersectionality* to describe the macro, structural perpetuations of systemic oppression, discrimination, and privilege that interact and manifest as health inequities and disparities.[9,10] A population's multidimensional, compounding identities and positionings (e.g., race, ethnicity, sex, gender, immigration status) are crucial to consider, as they simultaneously intersect. The extant vulnerable populations literature alludes to related themes (e.g., layers of marginalization, integrated vulnerability, heterogeneity) but falls short of naming intersectionality.[6,7] This omission demonstrates the necessity to embed intersectionality in vulnerable populations discourse. Integrating intersectionality with the concept of *vulnerabilized* situates individuals within their macrolevel contexts, acknowledges the interaction of multiple forms of marginalization, emphasizes the need for systemic accountability, and prioritizes structural interventions attuned to these complexities to advance health equity.[9]

Vulnerabilized shares similarities with commonly used verbiage but offers a linguistic shift to acknowledge the nexus of underlying, and often obscured, upstream determinants that shape vulnerability.[11] Critiques of the terminology currently used to describe vulnerable populations point to its paternalistic and oppressive undertones, investment in maintaining social control, and contribution to stigmatization and exclusion by way of labeling and blaming while disregarding populations' assets and agency.[8,12] A variety of terms are often erroneously used synonymously in the vulnerable populations literature without recognizing the risks of further perpetuating stigma, discrimination, inequity, and disparity.

The haphazard use and assumption of terms (e.g., *marginalized*, *hard to reach*, *underprivileged*) as interchangeable without consideration of their meaning risks oversimplifying complex, multidimensional concepts. For example, *marginalized* has become increasingly relied on to discuss populations burdened by health disparities when it might rather, more aptly, describe populations systemically pushed to the margins, or the periphery, who, as a result, have been vulnerabilized. Similarly, *hard to reach* has been employed to describe the perceived inaccessibility of populations without adequate acknowledgment of the role of marginalization in their distancing. These subtle, yet significant differences must be parsed out to avoid common pitfalls associated with misuse (e.g., exclusion, stigma).[8,12]

As public health practitioners, we have a responsibility to intentionally select our language, given our understanding of how language perpetuates social norms, influences attitudes, guides actions, and determines priorities. Given the limitations of our current lexicon, coupled with the potential harms of inaccurate or inadequate terminology, we call for attention to be devoted to the intentional use of precise, descriptive language when discussing vulnerabilized populations. It is the responsibility of the field to acknowledge and address the inadequacies and impacts of commonly used language in contributing to the adverse conditions from which we draw priorities. Therefore, we propose a transition away from a dependence on broad, seemingly catchall descriptors to the conscientious use of precise terms, such as *vulnerabilized*, when appropriate and meaningful to effectively communicate pertinent distinctions in our current vocabulary.

Additionally, public health efforts must first actively collaborate with communities being labeled to ensure that descriptors not only resonate but also empower and validate lived experiences. Motivations for labeling populations should be weighed against their implications and effects. Approaches that safeguard autonomy (e.g., person-first language, community-based participatory research) and ownership of personal narratives, identities, and experiences should be prioritized.

In conclusion, framing health equity with the term *vulnerabilized* recognizes that populations are not ambiguously vulnerable but rather are vulnerabilized, which more aptly positions us to address the root causes of health disparities. Failing to consider the power of language used to convey vulnerability inadequately holds accountable the systems that create and maintain inequities and disparities at the expense of the populations we serve. Regardless of whether *vulnerabilized* becomes a widely accepted term, the importance of using intentional language cannot be overstated. This is not merely a call for a semantic adjustment but also a reorientation toward social justice–based equity efforts, beginning with language.

Although we have made the case for *vulnerabilized*, it is our hope that this is not the end of the conversation but rather the beginning, motivating public health practitioners to intentionally choose their language, collaborate with those being labeled, and consider the impacts of the language chosen to describe populations. *Vulnerabilized* offers a perspective through which stakeholders, researchers, practitioners, and policymakers can better understand and address the systemic origins and evolving dynamics of vulnerability among individuals and populations. AJPH

CORRESPONDENCE

Correspondence should be sent to Camryn M. Garrett, 915 Greene St, Columbia, SC 29201 (e-mail: camrynmg@email.sc.edu). Reprints can be ordered at http://www.ajph.org by clicking the "Reprints" link.

PUBLICATION INFORMATION

Full Citation: Garrett CM, Altman R. Vulnerabilized: revisiting the language of the vulnerable populations framework. *Am J Public Health*. 2024;114(2): 177–179.

Acceptance Date: November 16, 2023.

DOI: https://doi.org/10.2105/AJPH.2023.307532

CONTRIBUTORS

The authors contributed equally to this editorial.

CONFLICTS OF INTEREST

The authors have no conflicts of interest to declare.

REFERENCES

1. Crear-Perry J, Correa-de-Araujo R, Lewis Johnson T, McLemore MR, Neilson E, Wallace M. Social and structural determinants of health inequities in maternal health. *J Womens Health (Larchmt)*. 2021;30(2):230–235. https://doi.org/10.1089/jwh.2020.8882
2. Levine C, Faden R, Grady C, Hammerschmidt D, Eckenwiler L, Sugarman J. A response to commentators on "The Limitations of 'Vulnerability' as a Protection for Human Research Participants." *Am J Bioeth*. 2004;4(3):W32. https://doi.org/10.1080/15265160490508954

3. US Department of Health and Human Services. Read the *Belmont Report*. January 15, 2018. Available at: https://www.hhs.gov/ohrp/regulations-and-policy/belmont-report/read-the-belmont-report/index.html. Accessed August 14, 2023.
4. Flaskerud JH, Winslow BJ. Conceptualizing vulnerable populations health-related research. *Nurs Res.* 1998;47(2):69–78. https://doi.org/10.1097/00006199-199803000-00005
5. Alberta Health Services. Towards an understanding of health equity: glossary. July 25, 2011. Available at: https://www.albertahealthservices.ca/poph/hi-poph-surv-shsa-tpgwg-glossary.pdf. Accessed December 19, 2023.
6. Walker AK, Fox EL. Why marginalization, not vulnerability, can best identify people in need of special medical and nutrition care. *AMA J Ethics.* 2018;20(10):E941–E947. https://doi.org/10.1001/amajethics.2018.941
7. Wolf S, Hinkel J, Hallier M, et al. Clarifying vulnerability definitions and assessments using formalisation. *Int J Clim Chang Strateg Manag.* 2013;5(1):54–70. https://doi.org/10.1108/17568691311299363
8. Brown K. "Vulnerability": handle with care. *Ethics Soc Welf.* 2011;5(3):313–321. https://doi.org/10.1080/17496535.2011.597165
9. Crenshaw K. Demarginalizing the intersection of race and sex: a Black feminist critique of antidiscrimination doctrine, feminist theory and antiracist politics. In: Maschke KJ, ed. *Feminist Legal Theories.* Abingdon, UK: Routledge; 1997:139–167.
10. Bowleg L. The problem with the phrase women and minorities: intersectionality—an important theoretical framework for public health. *Am J Public Health.* 2012;102(7):1267–1273. https://doi.org/10.2105/AJPH.2012.300750
11. Braveman P. What are health disparities and health equity? We need to be clear. *Public Health Rep.* 2014;129(suppl 2):5–8. https://doi.org/10.1177/00333549141291S203
12. Clark B, Preto N. Exploring the concept of vulnerability in health care. *CMAJ.* 2018;190(11):E308–E309. https://doi.org/10.1503/cmaj.180242

Public Health Preparedness Practitioners: Fluent in Disaster

Caleb Kuddes, BA

ABOUT THE AUTHOR

Caleb Kuddes is an emergency response coordinator at Douglas County Health Department, Omaha, NE, and a student at the College of Public Health, University of Nebraska Medical Center, Omaha.

See also The Languages of Public Health, pp. 164–192.

Many public health practitioners are multilingual; some are fluent in Spanish or Russian, others in Farsi or K'iche. Such professionals are invaluable in public health because their skills allow them to communicate across language barriers, uniting diverse publics into one public and streamlining the delivery of crucial services. Public health emergency preparedness (PHEP) practitioners, however, must be fluent in their own unique idiom: that of disaster.

Since 2002[1] PHEP has provided federal money to health departments to ensure preparedness for public health threats. PHEP prescribes 15 capabilities that a jurisdiction must fulfill to prepare for and respond to disasters and allows most health departments to maintain at least one staff member who works as a PHEP practitioner. These capabilities require practitioners to converse in scientific, medical, managerial, and sociological languages. Most, if not all, health departments also require the assistance of outside agencies to fulfill their PHEP capabilities, necessitating strong relationships with partners that have their own technical languages. Because of the requirements imposed on them by their grant, PHEP practitioners must be multilingual before disaster ever strikes, fluently interpreting public health theory and practice for and between coresponders and recovery agencies.

When disasters do strike, although one or few agencies may take a leading role, a successful response requires the coordination of many diverse entities. In the larger response structure, PHEP practitioners are often tasked with a leading position in addition to connecting their public health department to the response. As a public health emergency response coordinator, I served this dual role during the COVID-19 pandemic and often found myself having to understand not only different technical "languages" but even whole "language families."

Disaster response in the United States is practiced with a whole community approach, which incorporates local, state, and federal responders, nongovernmental organizations, and even unaffiliated individuals into a seamless and unified preparedness effort.[2] Although some organizations that work closely together, such as police and fire departments, speak in closely related terms akin to interrelated languages, the unique terminology of health care or disaster volunteer organizations are far less clear to the uninitiated.

In a previous career, I worked as a deputy sheriff and emergency dispatcher, which, in public health, helped me to communicate critical health information to first responders. Another responsibility that I had, however, was conducting epidemiological investigations. To a former law enforcement officer, interviewing and investigating came easy—the difficulty came when I realized that obtaining data was not the end. Patients who were ill, losing work, and isolated had needs more important than providing me with information. To grow in my role, I became active in my local Community Organizations Active in Disaster, which connected volunteer groups, ministerial organizations, and charities to the COVID-19 response. Over time, I learned that the broad mix of competencies required for PHEP practitioners to serve their communities allows them to bridge disciplinary gaps and translate terms, concepts, and methods across barriers. Like the traditionally multilingual public health practitioner, the PHEP professional can unite various response communities into one community, rendering the areas they serve more resilient, unified, and able to respond to disasters. Consequently, they should be incorporated into all emergency planning and response efforts.

Historically, this has not always been the case. One of the most important relationships PHEP practitioners must cultivate is with emergency management. Rose et al. write that public health agencies responded to disasters and complex emergencies long before civil defense was reorganized into modern emergency management, and for much of the respective histories of the disciplines, interactions between the two were rare.[3] Since the advent of all-hazards preparedness and PHEP, however, the objectives and responsibilities of public health and emergency management have increasingly dovetailed. The same holds true for other emergency and disaster response agencies.

Through joint responses, such as the responses to the COVID-19 pandemic and the 2001 Amerithrax attacks, public health departments have built strong relationships with the US military,[4] law enforcement,[5] fire, and emergency medical services agencies.[6] Grounded in public health, PHEP practitioners are trained in offering the 10 essential public health services, ensuring their facility with health science and objective data interpretation and centering all their work on equity.[7] This necessitates close relationships with organizations, both governmental and nongovernmental, that serve minority populations and those with access and functional needs. Finally, PHEP practitioners work closely with their local health care establishment, including hospital and nonhospital points of care, and their local health care coalition.

Because of the unique development of all these disciplines, coordination among them is not simply a question of ensuring that differing concepts are understood. Sometimes, it is akin to an act of translation. What graphemes are to a writing system, acronyms are to the languages of agencies involved in disaster response, and each discipline has its own unique roster: emergency managers discourse in JICs (Joint Information Centers), THIRAs (Threat and Hazard Identification and Risk Assessment), and the ICS (Incident Command System); whereas public health sets up PODs (Points of Dispensing) and writes CHAs (Community Health Assessments), and their corresponding CHIPs (Community Health Improvement Plans).

Perhaps no fact illustrates the proliferation of response acronyms better than the existence of the *FEMA Acronyms, Abbreviations and Terms* report, which catalogs 477 pages of acronyms currently in use.[8] During the COVID-19 pandemic, for example, I spent hours in meetings crammed with acronyms. Stakeholders as diverse as emergency management, meat processing facilities, schools and daycare facilities, and police and fire departments needed to learn from me as much as they could about the state of the pandemic, while simultaneously giving me the story of the pandemic from their perspectives as efficiently as possible.

In the language of disaster, that meant that we spoke in acronyms. The breakneck pace of meetings and jarringly quick guidance changes left little time to study—those of us who had much to learn had to learn quickly. Additionally, not only did this critical public health information flow laterally between stakeholders, I also had to translate it to promote action both up to leadership and elected officials and outward to the public, all of whom communicate in their own "dialect." Diverse communication needs also exist in disasters, in which public health serves a supporting role. In 2019, I participated in a response to devastating floods that required every responder to quickly gain facility with the language of emergency management. The health department representative, for example, was drafted to assist in directing people displaced by flooding to shelters under the supervision of the local shelter team. Every disaster response has unique needs, and PHEP practitioners must maintain enough linguistic flexibility to communicate in lead and support roles.

Disaster response, like traditional public health work, requires facility with many languages, as well as the ability to translate and interpret them for others. In the wake of the COVID-19 pandemic, PHEP practitioners are more necessary than ever, because they, unique among disaster responders, are fluent in all the languages necessary to connect response and recovery, theory and practice. They are the bridge between public health and the disaster response ecosystem but offer value even beyond that connection. Fluent in all dialects of disaster, they should be incorporated ever more firmly into the larger emergency preparedness and response community. AJPH

CORRESPONDENCE

Correspondence should be sent to Caleb Kuddes, 1585 Highway 275, Fremont, NE 68025 (e-mail: ckuddes@unmc.edu). Reprints can be ordered at http://www.ajph.org by clicking the "Reprints" link.

PUBLICATION INFORMATION

Full Citation: Kuddes C. Public health preparedness practitioners: fluent in disaster. *Am J Public Health*. 2024;114(2):180–182.

Acceptance Date: November 16, 2023.

DOI: https://doi.org/10.2105/AJPH.2023.307533

ACKNOWLEDGMENTS

Thank you to Keith Hansen, Sharon Medcalf, Constantine Sarsamă, and Peter Winsky, who read this editorial and provided suggestions.

CONFLICTS OF INTEREST

The author has no conflicts of interest to disclose.

REFERENCES

1. Murthy BP, Molinari N-AM, LeBlanc TT, Vagi SJ, Avchen RN. Progress in public health emergency preparedness—United States, 2001–2016. *Am J Public Health*. 2017;107(suppl 2):S180–S185. https://doi.org/10.2105/AJPH.2017.304038
2. US Department of Homeland Security, Federal Emergency Management Agency. A whole community approach to emergency management:

principles, themes, and pathways for action. Available at: https://www.fema.gov/sites/default/files/2020-07/whole_community_dec2011__2.pdf. Accessed December 10, 2023.

3. Rose DA, Murthy S, Brooks J, Bryant J. The evolution of public health emergency management as a field of practice. *Am J Public Health*. 2017;107(suppl 2):S126–S133. https://doi.org/10.2105/AJPH.2017.303947
4. Dumproff JB, Bishara J, Copeland N, Fredricks T. Integrating US National Guard with public health partners at COVID-19 testing sites in West Virginia counties with high rural and minority populations: lessons learned. *Health Secur*. 2022;20(1):58–64. https://doi.org/10.1089/hs.2021.0082
5. Butler JC, Cohen ML, Friedman CR, Scripp RM, Watz CG. Collaboration between public health and law enforcement: new paradigms and partnerships for bioterrorism planning and response. *Emerg Infect Dis*. 2002;8(10):1152–1156. https://doi.org/10.3201/eid0810.020400
6. Al Amiry A, Maguire BJ. Emergency medical services (EMS) calls during COVID-19: early lessons learned for systems planning (a narrative review). *Open Access Emerg Med*. 2021;13:407–414. https://doi.org/10.2147/OAEM.S324568
7. Public Health Accreditation Board. The ten essential public health services. 2023. Available at: https://phaboard.org/center-for-innovation/public-health-frameworks/the-10-essential-public-health-services. Accessed December 10, 2023.
8. US Department of Homeland Security, Federal Emergency Management Agency. *FEMA Acronyms, Abbreviations and Terms*. Available at: https://www.fema.gov/sites/default/files/documents/fema-acronyms-abbreviations-terms_FAAT_03-2023.pdf. Accessed December 10, 2023.

Medical Etymology: A Journey of Identity

Campbell Mitchell, BA

ABOUT THE AUTHOR

Campbell Mitchell is with the Yale School of Public Health, New Haven, CT.

See also The Languages of Public Health, pp. 164–192.

When I was young, I was diagnosed with "juvenile diabetes mellitus." My new medical team invested time and empathy to try to give my bewildered parents and myself the most comprehensive education possible. They explained not only the steps that we needed to take for me to survive and live a full life, but also the underlying science. I learned many new concepts this way that are still relevant to me as a public health student: concepts like etiology, risk factors, and intervention trials. My big question, however, went initially unanswered. What was the shape and essence of this thing that required me to upend my life on pain of death?

This is never an easy question. Although most new research at that time described type 1 diabetes mellitus as an autoimmune disease, this was still regarded as one working hypothesis among many. My team continuously reiterated that I had done nothing wrong and had no reason to feel ashamed. Yet in absence of some other way to contextualize the problem, I couldn't help but doubt.

At a follow-up, my endocrinologist asked me if I knew what I had. I responded as I had been taught: "juvenile diabetes mellitus." He asked if I knew what that meant. I said that I knew "juvenile" meant young, but the rest was lost on me. He explained with a mischievous smile that the words diabetes mellitus came from the ancient Greeks and referred to an old diagnostic of tasting urine; diabetes mellitus describes someone whose urine tastes sweet, which we now know is because it has sugar in it.

This tidbit of context allowed me to face my diagnosis with laughter rather than terror. But deeper than this, understanding the etymology gave me context that this wasn't some unknown monster that had attacked me alone; on the contrary, there was a whole archeological record. Scholars of a bygone age had picked a name based on what they could observe and understand, and civilization had kept working the problem until eventually it became survivable. The accepted jargon was gradually changing to be more in line with modern evidence and practice, which reflected an accelerating improvement in both our current abilities and our hope for the future.

The language of health, and specifically medicine and academia, is usually constructed by experts to communicate with other experts; as in the case of diabetes, it often draws on Latin and Greek, the historical languages of the educated elite. It is an easy target for critique because of its inscrutability to the lay person, despite its professional utility.

Nevertheless, I submit that when contextualized appropriately, jargon can enhance interventions for both professionals and laypeople. Understanding the linguistic heritage of my diagnosis helped me synthesize the education provided by my team and find a place in support communities. Language can become the focal point for organization and advocacy. The Juvenile Diabetes Research Foundation persists, despite "type 1" having largely replaced "juvenile" as the medically preferred term, because the linguistic heritage has been embraced by a community of advocates.

My lesson as a student in public health is that professional language is not exclusively mine but is the shared heritage of all those whose lives and identities my work affects. I have an obligation to be a good steward in my own usage, and to share the context with those who might benefit from such education. With a growing body of evidence supporting community support as a determinant of health, using language not only to avoid isolating, but to actively empower, becomes all the more important for public health practitioners. AJPH

CORRESPONDENCE

Correspondence should be sent to Campbell Mitchell, Yale School of Public Health, 60 College St, New Haven, CT 06520-8034 (e-mail: campbell.mitchell@yale.edu). Reprints can be ordered at http://www.ajph.org by clicking the "Reprints" link.

PUBLICATION INFORMATION

Full Citation: Mitchell C. Medical etymology: a journey of identity. *Am J Public Health*. 2024; 114(2):183.

Acceptance Date: November 16, 2023

DOI: https://doi.org/10.2105/AJPH.2023.307535

CONFLICTS OF INTEREST

The author has no conflicts of interest to disclose.

One Afternoon at a Vaccination Clinic

Faith E. Muller, BSN, RN

ABOUT THE AUTHOR

Faith E. Muller is an MPH student in the Department of Public and Community Health, Liberty University, Lynchburg, VA.

See also The Languages of Public Health, pp. 164–192.

Multiple languages in a cross-cultural space can lead to confusion, mixed public health messages, and even barriers to health. The Bible states, "Therefore, if I do not know the meaning of the language, I shall be a foreigner to him who speaks, and he who speaks will be a foreigner to me" (1 Corinthians 14:11). I have seen this in public health. While participating in a pediatric vaccine drive run by my local health department, I encountered multiple communication-based barriers to public health in a single afternoon and witnessed the importance of a culturally and linguistically competent workforce.

When caring for a Filipino patient that afternoon, I noticed his mandatory Vaccine Information Statement (VIS) was in Spanish. One of the 10 Essential Public Health Services is to educate and inform through communication.[1] Researchers[2,3] recognize the VIS as an important tool for increasing health literacy and improving vaccination rates; it is a critical element in educating patients and their parents. When I realized the patient's VIS was in Spanish, I notified the staff worker performing check-in and asked for an English VIS. The staff worker insisted the patient needed a Spanish sheet. I explained that he was from the Philippines, not Latin America, but she did not believe me. In one final attempt to convince her that he needed an English VIS, I asked him in Spanish if he spoke Spanish. He looked at me with hooded eyes and raised eyebrows, and stated, "I have no idea what you just said." The staff worker was still skeptical but reluctantly agreed to give him an additional VIS in English. I wondered how many Filipino children went home that day with an indecipherable VIS, missing out on an important (and mandated[3]) opportunity for health education.

My last patient that afternoon was brought to me by an administrator of the elementary school hosting the clinic. He ushered two boys to my table and stated that the older brother would translate. I had previously vaccinated the older brother, and he knew I could speak Spanish. The older brother began speaking to me in Spanish, but the administrator interrupted him. "No, speak in English! He can speak in English," he stated as an aside to me. Despite the insistence and multiple urgings of the administrator, the older brother refused to speak to me in English, and we completed everything in Spanish.

Schwalbe[4] writes that language is more than communication of facts. Language is emotional, and it helps us connect to our identity. Zhao et al.[5] found that utilizing health care services is stressful for linguistic minorities. Additionally, communicating in a second language led to an unwillingness to access health care. Needing to communicate in a second language when accessing health care can lead to a decreased usage of health services, which in turn can exacerbate existing health disparities.[5] A linguistically diverse workforce[1] is vital to promoting "equitable access" (another essential service).

Communication is indispensable for public health. In the microcosm of an afternoon vaccination clinic, I saw language issues reveal barriers to public health, and I saw that without a linguistically diverse staff, essential public health services suffer. Providing education in cultural competence and hiring linguistically diverse staff are two practical steps that local health departments can take to improve access to public health. As the number of speakers of other languages in the United States increases, and communities become more diverse, we must learn to identify and be aware of the cultures and preferred languages of the populations we are serving, and we must promote a linguistically diverse and culturally competent public health workforce to decrease health disparities. AJPH

CORRESPONDENCE

Correspondence should be sent to Faith E. Muller, BSN, RN, Online Graduate Student, Liberty University, Department of Public and Community Health, 1971 University Blvd, Lynchburg, VA 24515 (e-mail: femuller@liberty.edu). Reprints can be ordered at http://www.ajph.org by clicking the "Reprints" link.

PUBLICATION INFORMATION

Full Citation: Muller FE. One afternoon at a vaccination clinic. *Am J Public Health*. 2024;114(2): 184–185.

Acceptance Date: November 16, 2023.

DOI: https://doi.org/10.2105/AJPH.2023.307536

CONFLICTS OF INTEREST

The author has no conflicts of interest to disclose.

REFERENCES

1. Centers for Disease Control and Prevention. Ten essential public health services. Updated March 6, 2023. Available at: https://www.cdc.gov/publichealthgateway/publichealthservices/essentialhealthservices.html. Accessed August 25, 2023.
2. Constable C, Chapman CR. Bolstering trust in the human papillomavirus vaccine through improved communication in the Vaccine Information Statement. *Vaccine*. 2019;37(31):4241–4242. https://doi.org/10.1016/j.vaccine.2019.05.094
3. Jacobs AT, Macintosh JLB, Luthy KE, Beckstrand RL, Robinson MS, Macintosh CI. Parental reports of Vaccine Information Statement usage in Utah. *J Am Assoc Nurse Pract*. 2023;35(5):299–305. https://doi.org/10.1097/JXX.0000000000000845
4. Schwalbe DM. In the language of their hearts: emotions and language choice in child–parent interaction, insights from a Yupik village. *Etud Inuit*. 2021;45(1/2):171–206. https://www.jstor.org/stable/27136423
5. Zhao Y, Segalowitz N, Voloshyn A, Chamoux E, Ryder AG. Language barriers to healthcare for linguistic minorities: the case of second language-specific health communication anxiety. *Health Commun*. 2021;36(3):334–346. https://doi.org/10.1080/10410236.2019.1692488

When Public Health Terms Become Vernacular

Nishita J. Matangi, MPH

ABOUT THE AUTHOR

Nishita J. Matangi is with the School of Public Health and School of Behavioral Health, Loma Linda University, Loma Linda, CA.

See also The Languages of Public Health, pp. 164–192.

Winter 2020. I was a second-year Master of Public Health student anticipating graduation while working in my school's communications office incorporating public health education into social media content. I remember having conversations with friends and family about a novel virus in East Asia. Within a few weeks, coronavirus and COVID-19 dominated the headlines of every local and global news platform with talks of the "curve" and needing to flatten said curve. Many changed their profile pictures on social media to include the "flatten the curve" frame. Epidemiological terms quickly became popular vernacular. The top Google searches were related to the virus.[1] A few months before, public health was a rare or misunderstood term; however, by spring, conversations surrounding disease transmission and incubation periods were normal for the general public.

As a part of our media strategy, the communication office created a series of videos that explained the terms used and addressed concerns being discussed in the news. Our first video was titled "What exactly is the curve and why should we flatten it?" This was followed by several short videos about epidemiology, how viruses and germs work, and effective ways to disinfect. All these videos used academic public health terminology but were explained in laypersons' terms and delivered in a conversational format to minimize the distance between academia and the population and promote accessibility and learning. As a result, we saw a 1205% increase in engagement, a 47.3% increase in net audience, and a 436.5% increase in video views. Through this experience, I concluded that there is no issue with including public health terms in public messaging if there is a reasonable effort to explain the terms in a relevant and relatable way to the target audience.

A balance between health education and accessibility is imperative when creating public health content for communities. Education creates opportunities for self-advocacy. Being able to make informed decisions concerning an individual's health and the health of their family should be a basic right. But advocacy requires knowledge.[2] Having the appropriate language allows them to better converse with their providers, ask better questions, and make more informed decisions.

On the other hand, it is our responsibility as professionals to make these conversations accessible by creating content that is appropriate for the target audience by addressing factors like language, reading level, and cultural relevance.[3] Although the public health community prioritized education at the start of the pandemic, as the influx of information increased, messaging became less clear. This increased the risk for misinformation, which was exemplified when vaccines entered the global and national conversation. The term mRNA was introduced without appropriate education, resulting in public fear. Although it was a basic term for the research and medical community, it was new to the average person and incited fear.[4]

The evolution of the use of public health terms during the pandemic and since then has significantly shaped conversations on social media, making an urgent case for the need for research on equitable access to health information. I have recognized through firsthand experience not only the need for appropriate health education and promotion but also the significance of organizational health literacy to shift the burden of equitable health information from the consumer to content creators like government and community organizations as well as health and academic institutions.[5] We have learned much from our collective pandemic experience. Those lessons should be applied in everyday public health to regain and maintain the public's trust. We must be prepared to create content that the public is able to clearly receive when the next pandemic or emergency unfolds.[6] AJPH

CORRESPONDENCE

Correspondence should be sent to Nishita J. Matangi, 24951 Circle Dr, Loma Linda, CA 92354 (e-mail: nmatangi@llu.edu). Reprints can be ordered at https://ajph.org by clicking the "Reprints" link.

PUBLICATION INFORMATION

Full Citation: Matangi NJ. When public health terms become vernacular. *Am J Public Health.* 2024;114(2):186–187.

Acceptance Date: November 16, 2023.

DOI: https://doi.org/10.2105/AJPH.2023.307538

ACKNOWLEDGMENTS

Thank you to the Communications Office and Practicum Office at Loma Linda University School of Public Health for considering and implementing this project.

CONFLICTS OF INTEREST

There are no conflicts of interest to report.

REFERENCES

1. Google Trends. Coronavirus search trends. Available at: https://trends.google.com/trends/story/GB_cu_JSW_pHABAADqAM_en. Accessed October 8, 2023.
2. Schmidt EK, Faieta J, Tanner K. Scoping review of self-advocacy education interventions to improve care. *OTJR (Thorofare N J)*. 2020;40(1):50–56. https://doi.org/10.1177/1539449219860583
3. Communicate Health. *A Framework for Equity-Centered Health Communication*. 2023. Available at: https://communicatehealth.com/wp-content/uploads/CH-ECHC-Framework.pdf. Accessed October 8, 2023.
4. Rzymski P, Borkowski L, Drag M, et al. The strategies to support the COVID-19 vaccination with evidence-based communication and tackling misinformation. *Vaccines (Basel)*. 2021;9(2):109. https://doi.org/10.3390/vaccines9020109
5. Palumbo R, Annarumma C. The importance of being health literate: an organizational health literacy approach. In: *Excellence in Services International Conference*. Liverpool, England: John Moores University; 2014: 247–262.
6. Ataguba OA, Ataguba JE. Social determinants of health: the role of effective communication in the COVID-19 pandemic in developing countries. *Glob Health Action*. 13(1):1788263. https://doi.org/10.1080/16549716.2020.1788263

Imagery as a Participatory Tool of Resilience for Marginalized Persons

Grace Iona A. Adan, MPH

ABOUT THE AUTHOR

Grace Iona A. Adan is a DrPh candidate at the School of Public Health, University at Albany, State University of New York, Albany.

See also The Languages of Public Health, pp. 164–192.

The transformation of global population health in recent decades has led to growing interest in inclusion and empowerment for marginalized individuals. As students whose contributions to the field will shape research and advocacy, we must prioritize participatory engagement. A culture of active listening motivates public health professionals to amplify the voices of individuals whose circumstances encourage suboptimal mental well-being or physical health. One's exposure to the societal contagions of religious minority oppression, ableism, sexism, racism, transphobia, homophobia, xenophobia, and colorism diminishes health-related quality of life. Through an examination of how the term "marginalized" shapes our work, we gain insights into fostering visibility through storytelling for individuals affected by adversity.

Individuals who are marginalized are "relegated to a marginal position within a society or group,"[1] which connotes a de facto hierarchy characterized by power imbalances and social exclusion. In conversational English, a "margin" denotes some outermost spatial boundary beyond the scope of the mainstream or some predominant majority. As noted by medical ethics scholars, classification of the oft-synonymous term "vulnerability" is difficult to standardize but is defined by one's susceptibility to threats of harm.[2] The adage "a picture is worth a thousand words" allows us to consider how image capture evokes an alternative expression of language for those living among us who incur limited social capital.

As public health practitioners in training, our imperative should be to move the goalpost of community engagement beyond the traditional arena of spoken communication. Intracommunity relationships may be present that undermine marginalized residents, whereby their voice is silenced because of isolation in the collective group. Social vulnerability among marginalized members of society is expressed by persons with lived experience through focus groups, engagement workshops, and listening session town halls.[3] Photovoice has emerged as a tool that enables one to illustrate community characteristics related to the built environment, housing, and physical hazards using photography.[4] Photographs provide an opportunity for meaningful agency among marginalized persons, who may be reticent to seek out available community supports or are unaware of local resources.

Our pursuit of idea exchange as community public health workers should not be restricted to conversational dialogue, as we can learn from marginalized residents through themes displayed in collaborative photovoice initiatives. When we serve communities, through public or private sector disease prevention programs, the work of public health contributes to improved social cohesion. Our work should incorporate sustainable relationship building to encourage marginalized persons to engage with health promotion and surveillance activities. Self-reflection toward implicit and conscious biases requires introspective awareness of our own stature as health professionals who benefit from privilege and power.[5] However, we may not realize that our altruistic intentions cannot guarantee trust building with those who are wary of institutionalized health services. Transparency is enhanced when we acknowledge available (or nonexistent) community assets that are highlighted by photographic renderings to improve health outcomes.

A disenfranchised position in society does not presume permanency throughout one's life. Public health achievements are a proxy outcome of social justice reform efforts that identify social patterns that serve to diminish the health playing field of marginalized populations.[6] Tailored interventions that solicit ongoing feedback from our underserved end users using an accessible variety of communication modalities can help circumvent barriers to parity. To counteract a culture of historically cyclical ignorance of the needs of at-risk communities, our work should be cross-sectoral. Interdisciplinary coalition building with advocates, nonprofit agencies, and governmental human services stakeholders is of paramount importance to health justice for all. As we aim to sustain such partnerships,

AJPH February 2024, Vol. 114, No. 2

our marginalized neighbors should be emboldened to vocalize their life course perspectives pictorially through self-selected photographs *and* verbally through written or spoken means. AJPH

CORRESPONDENCE

Correspondence should be sent to Grace Iona Abby Adan, Department of Health Policy, Management, & Behavior, 1 University Place, Edward & Frances George Education Center, Rensselaer, NY 12144 (e-mail: gjama-adan@albany.edu). Reprints can be ordered at http://www.ajph.org by clicking the "Reprints" link.

PUBLICATION INFORMATION

Full Citation: Adan GIA. Imagery as a participatory tool of resilience for marginalized persons. *Am J Public Health*. 2024;114(2):188–189.

Acceptance Date: November 18, 2023.

DOI: https://doi.org/10.2105/AJPH.2023.307534

CONFLICTS OF INTEREST

The author has no conflicts of interest to declare.

REFERENCES

1. *Merriam-Webster*. S.v. "marginalized (adj.)." August 16, 2023. Available at: https://www.merriam-webster.com/dictionary/marginalized. Accessed August 22, 2023.
2. Wrigley A, Dawson A. Vulnerability and marginalized populations. In: Barrett DH, Ortmann LW, Dawson A, Saenz C, Reis A, Bolan G, eds. *Public Health Ethics: Cases Spanning the Globe*. Cham, Switzerland: Springer; 2016. https://doi.org/10.1007/978-3-319-23847-0_7
3. Luchenski S, Maguire N, Aldridge RW, et al. What works in inclusion health: overview of effective interventions for marginalised and excluded populations. *Lancet*. 2018;391(10117):266–280. https://doi.org/10.1016/S0140-6736(17)31959-1
4. Wang C, Burris MA. Photovoice: concept, methodology, and use for participatory needs assessment. *Health Educ Behav*. 1997;24(3):369–387. https://doi.org/10.1177/109019819702400309
5. Beech BM, Ford C, Thorpe RJ Jr, Bruce MA, Norris KC. Poverty, racism, and the public health crisis in America. *Front Public Health*. 2021;9:699049. https://doi.org/10.3389/fpubh.2021.699049
6. Galea S, Vaughan RD. Public health and marginalized populations: a public health of consequence, October 2019. *Am J Public Health*. 2019;109(10):1327–1328. https://doi.org/10.2105/AJPH.2019.305293

Unseen and Unheard: Increasing the Visibility of Limited English Proficiency Individuals Through a Language Justice Framework

Tashfia Jilu, BA

ABOUT THE AUTHOR

Tashfia Jilu is a dual master's student at the School of Public Health and School of Social Work, University of Michigan, Ann Arbor.

See also The Languages of Public Health, pp. 164–192.

AJPH February 2024, Vol. 114, No. 2

Recently, I received a text from my mom asking how to describe her symptom—*"amar haath paa chabay"*—in English. Literally, this means "my hands and feet are chewing," but I knew the translation had to make sense in a medical context. After a few minutes of deliberating on the feelings evoked by various English words, I decided the closest translation was "my hands and feet are throbbing." As a daughter of Bangladeshi immigrants, being an on-call interpreter was not new. Although my parents are now very comfortable speaking English, there are still times they need help finding just the right words to describe what they want to say.

Many children of immigrants living in the United States share the experience of growing up as interpreters and translators for their limited English proficient (LEP) parents. LEP refers to "individuals who do not speak English as their primary language and have a limited ability to read, speak, write, or understand English."[1] According to 2013 US census data, 25.4 million Americans identified as having limited English proficiency,[2] a number that continues to grow.

Growing up, the primary language spoken in our household was Sylheti, a dialect of Bangla, which allowed my siblings and me to become fluent in Bangla. The significance of us learning our mother tongue is particularly noteworthy given the history of Bangladesh. During Bangladesh's fight for independence and liberation from West Pakistan, one of the most renowned campaigns was the language movement against the declaration of Urdu as the official state language. During a protest in 1952, five university students were murdered and thousands more injured.[3] Since then, February 21 has been celebrated in Bangladesh as Shohid Dibosh, Language Martyrs' Day. Yet, although some fought and died for the right to speak Bangla, US cultural structures are restricting the Bangladeshi community from using their mother tongue by forcing them to speak English to achieve an adequate quality of life.

In the United States, a person's ability to speak English well is crucial to obtain many, if not all, essential services. Getting a good education, being able to afford housing and transportation, engaging in civic life—these are difficult to achieve even for those who speak English. Not speaking English proficiently is an additional obstacle. It is inarguable, then, that language itself is an essential social determinant of health. Although language falls under the "social and community context" domain of social determinants of health, it tends to receive little attention in research, practice, and policy.

As with most structures of inequality, those of us who speak the dominant language seldom recognize it for the privilege that it is. My interest in the connection between language accessibility and health began when Anthony Hatch, PhD, a former professor, asked, "Whose voices are being left out of the conversations in public health? Whose untold stories are you going to tell?" These questions led me to conduct an undergraduate research study exploring language in health care and launched my academic trajectory toward public health.

My study focused on language services for LEP Bangladeshi patients and their lived experiences accessing health care in the United States. This project deepened my understanding of the importance of language in public health practice. I was able to better understand the need for dialect-specific interpreters, increased training in cultural and language humility for health care providers, and improving available language services. I conducted a notable interview during my study with an older man who described his challenges with language before a planned surgery:

> When they gave me instructions for preparing for the surgery, they gave them both in English and Bangla. However . . . the translation doesn't match up with what I was told by the doctor. . . . And I've mentioned before that the translations aren't accurate. . . . They just tell me that they use whatever they get [online] because they don't know how else to translate it.

The inaccurate translation provided to this patient could have led to severe medical consequences. Language evolves with people, their movements, and their thoughts. Language is ever changing, but online translating services use code that remains unchanged until someone intentionally updates it. We cannot rely on code to communicate with people.

Because of this combination of research-driven data and my own lived experiences, I have found that it is critical to incorporate the framework of language justice in public health. This framework is "based on the notion of respecting every individual's fundamental language rights—to be able to communicate, understand, and be understood in the language in which they prefer and feel most articulate and powerful."[4] Language provides the words and meanings that form culture, identity, and power, so researchers need to combine the language justice framework with intersectional frameworks to understand the lived experiences of LEP immigrants living in the United States.

Just as Bangladeshis cannot be separated from their historical fight for independence, language cannot be separated from historical context, lived experiences, and social embodiment. In her book *Archives of Tongues*, sociologist Moon Charania says, "Tongues reveal that language itself is an intensification of bodily capacity . . . these speech acts of flesh . . . are tightly entangled with racialized, classed, gendered, and sexualized ways of being in the world."[5(p19)] A language justice framework is integral for analyzing these intersectional facets of language and society.

Several immediate steps can be taken in public health practice to improve the experiences of the LEP population across different cultures and ethnicities living in the United States. One step is to standardize asking about preferred language when collecting demographic information from patients, clients, and community members. Community and government organizations can then use these data to provide tailored translations by employing community champions who understand linguistic and cultural nuances, rather than relying on online platforms that are often inaccurate.

Public health research can integrate the language justice framework to develop creative and community-engaged methods to collaborate with LEP communities and increase the research and evaluation needed to establish proper language services. One action step is to involve community champions, stakeholders, and LEP community members from the outset in research advisory boards and the design process. Another step is to be intentional and make space for research team members to reflect on their language privilege and its impact on study procedures.

I remember feeling frustration and stress for my mom that morning. A wrong translation could mean inaccurate diagnosis or prescription. What would have occurred had I not been there to help? Many LEP individuals will not have such easy access to an interpreter. Although focused on the Bangladeshi community, this editorial has broader implications for language and immigrant health research, as it addresses the need for accurate, culturally appropriate translations and emphasizes community-engaged participatory research for all LEP communities. To continue amplifying the voices of minorities, to allow them to be seen and heard, we must use language justice to focus efforts on one of the most fundamental aspects of public health and health care: language. AJPH

CORRESPONDENCE

Correspondence should be sent to Tashfia Jilu, 1415 Washington Heights, School of Public Health, Health Behavior and Health Education, University of Michigan, Ann Arbor, MI 48109 (e-mail: tjilu@umich.edu). Reprints can be ordered at http://www.ajph.org by clicking the "Reprints" link.

PUBLICATION INFORMATION

Full Citation: Jilu T. Unseen and unheard: increasing the visibility of limited English proficiency individuals through a language justice framework. *Am J Public Health*. 2024;114(2):190–192.

Acceptance Date: November 17, 2023.

DOI: https://doi.org/10.2105/AJPH.2023.307537

ACKNOWLEDGMENTS

I wish to express my sincere appreciation to Anthony Hatch, PhD, whose unwavering support and mentorship over the course of the past four years have been invaluable to my personal and academic growth. Additionally, my gratitude extends to Mary Janevic, PhD, MPH, and Paul Fleming, PhD, MPH, for their assistance in editing this editorial and guiding me through the intricacies of the publishing process. Most of all, I extend my deepest thanks to my parents, whose boundless kindness and unwavering support have been instrumental in shaping my character. I aspire to emulate their virtues and, above all, strive to make them proud.

CONFLICTS OF INTEREST

The author has no conflicts of interest to disclose.

REFERENCES

1. LEP.gov. Commonly asked questions and answers regarding limited English proficient (LEP) individuals. April 2011. Available at: https://www.lep.gov/sites/lep/files/media/document/2020-03/042511_QA_LEP_General_0.pdf. Accessed August 20, 2023.
2. US Census Bureau. Detailed languages spoken at home and ability to speak English for the population 5 years and over: 2009–2013. December 16, 2021. Available at: https://www.census.gov/data/tables/2013/demo/2009-2013-lang-tables.html. Accessed August 20, 2023.
3. Hamid H. Remembering the martyrs of the "Bengali Language Movement." February 18, 2019. Available at: https://www.sadf.eu/remembering-the-martyrs-of-the-bengali-language-movement. Accessed August 20, 2023.
4. Payton C, Lee J, Mercado APN, Uliasz A. Language justice during COVID-19. May 13, 2020. Available at: https://www.americanbar.org/groups/young_lawyers/about/initiatives/disaster-legal-services/language-justice-during-covid-19. Accessed August 20, 2023.
5. Charania M. *Archives of Tongues: An Intimate History of Brownness.* Durham, NC: Duke University Press; 2023.

From Farms to Pharma: A "Natural" History of Vaccine Production and Vaccine Skepticism

Tess Lanzarotta, PhD

See also Colgrove, p. 155.

In the era of synthetic biology, vaccine skeptics have made claims that vaccines are "unnatural," that the technology used to develop them is risky and untested, and that "naturally acquired" immunity is superior to vaccination. Public health practitioners and physicians alike have attempted to respond to these concerns by reminding patients and the public that vaccines generate a "natural" immune response. These negotiations over the language to describe vaccines are nothing new.

This article puts the relationship between vaccines and concepts like "nature" and "natural" in historical perspective. In the mid- to late 19th century, the smallpox vaccine, then the only vaccine available, was propagated on farms. Vaccine farmers—usually enterprising physicians—kept herds of cattle infected with cowpox, cultivating the virus "stock" from which the vaccine was derived.

By exploring how vaccine farmers established and maintained public confidence in their products, we can see that debates over vaccine safety have always involved concerted efforts to persuade the public to place their trust in technologies that might at first seem novel, strange, or even dangerous. More broadly, this article encourages readers to think about the shifting valences of the category "natural," particularly in a public health context. (*Am J Public Health*. 2024;114(2):193–201. https://doi.org/10.2105/AJPH.2023.307508)

Opponents of vaccination argue that "natural" immunity acquired through infection with disease is superior to the "artificial" immunity produced by vaccines. Organizations that spread vaccine misinformation have also stoked public fears that the COVID-19 vaccine is particularly dangerous because it is "unnatural" or "synthetic."[1] These ideas seem to be making an impact. Data suggest that some parents are hesitant to vaccinate young children against COVID-19 because of the perceived novelty of the vaccine and the technologies used to create it.[2] Many parents who reject vaccines also have a preoccupation with the "natural body," "natural living," and "natural childbirth." As sociologist Jennifer A. Reich points out, public health messaging that emphasizes that vaccines produce a "natural immune response" is a tactful response to these concerns. But such efforts can do little to address parents' broader concern that they live in a world full of dangerous, invisible, or unnatural toxins and chemicals.[3] Concerns about whether the substances that enter our bodies are "unnatural" are not limited to vaccines, but they are uniquely important when applied to a technology that requires widespread adoption to be maximally effective.

Anxieties surrounding corruption and pollution, of both bodies and vaccines, have animated debates over vaccination since its inception. For many in the 19th century, when vaccination first became widespread, the practice seemed to compromise bodily integrity by introducing dangerous foreign matter into the bloodstream.[4] Those who opposed vaccination argued that it was fundamentally "unnatural" or even "impious to engraft upon a Christian the diseases of a brute."[5] But, those who promoted vaccination emphasized its connections with both the laws of nature and the natural world. They framed vaccination as a "singular Gift of Providence" that represented God's will, rather than defying it.[6] They insisted that it was far safer than

AJPH February 2024, Vol. 114, No. 2

contracting "inoculated smallpox" or "natural cowpox."[7] And they also sought to associate the practice with pastoral or rural spaces, which symbolized health and vitality in the 19th-century imagination.

Vaccines, then, have not always been seen as particularly scientific or technological products. In the 19th century, terms like "nature," "natural," and "unnatural" were moving targets, and they remain so today. Their definitions are plural and fluctuate over time. This history is a source of both caution and hope. On one hand, specific and historically contingent definitions of "natural" and "unnatural" have been a feature of debates over the safety of vaccines are unlikely to ever fully disappear. On the other hand, vaccine producers and promoters have been successful in adapting their language to persuade people to undergo vaccination. This, too, seems unlikely to change.

FROM ARMS TO FARMS

In 1798, English physician Edward Jenner published *An Inquiry Into the Causes and Effects of the Variolæ Vaccinæ*, which demonstrated that exposure to cowpox could generate immunity to smallpox in humans. He had learned about the protective power of cowpox from dairy maids and tested it on a series of human subjects.[8] News of Jenner's discovery quickly spread around the world, as did the vaccine. Initially, the arm-to-arm method was the most popular. Physicians would administer cowpox scabs or dried pus into a lancet incision, wait until the patient had an inflamed lesion, and then transfer pus from one patient to another.[9] While many physicians on both sides of the Atlantic embraced vaccination and became involved in governmental efforts to centralize vaccine supplies, others began to express doubts. Physicians disagreed about whether the smallpox vaccine conferred lifelong immunity and debated whether a person needed medical training to safely perform vaccinations. In the United States, these arguments contributed to the wholesale abandonment in the 1820s of efforts to maintain a vaccine supply at the federal level.[10]

By the mid-19th century, more serious concerns about vaccination had emerged. For instance, in England, efforts to enforce compulsory vaccination were met with immediate resistance. Parents were concerned that arm-to-arm vaccination could spread "cancer, syphilis, scrofula, or mental illness," and that it constituted a form of "blood pollution" that was "unChristian."[11] In the United States, the problem was initially one of supply, rather than resistance. During the Civil War, when the Confederate and Union armies began to experience severe smallpox outbreaks, both tried to stop the spread of the disease with mass vaccination campaigns.[12] However, the vaccine was in short supply, and there were many reports of "spurious" or inactive vaccine matter and syphilis transmission. Most gruesomely, men who were already sick or malnourished sometimes developed gangrene and other secondary infections at vaccination sites.[13] By the 1870s, American medical journals acknowledged that arm-to-arm vaccination could spread illness.[14] The war, then, had a mixed legacy. It left Americans both more aware of the need for vaccination and more cognizant of its potential risks.[15]

Those who supported vaccination struggled to secure a vaccine supply and restore public trust in the practice. But they also looked for creative ways to mitigate the risks of vaccination. In 1840, an Italian physician named Giuseppe Negri began maintaining his vaccine supply within a herd of infected cattle, instead of relying on human hosts. It was not until the 1860s, after a medical conference in Lyon, France, that physicians outside of Italy learned of Negri's method. While they were impressed, there was some suspicion about the quality of the "Neapolitan 'stock' of virus." Some feared that it was the result of "retro-vaccine," a technique that involved vaccinating cows with vaccine matter harvested from infected humans. Many physicians believed that this technique was unsafe or ineffective.[16] To avoid potential contamination, doctors professed the need for a source of vaccine that was "purely and exclusively animal."[17] Negri's "stock" might not have spread far, but his ideas did, and they would soon revolutionize vaccine production.[18]

In 1866, a French doctor named Jean DePaul, who was the director of vaccination services for the Paris Academy of Medicine, reported a "spontaneous case" of cowpox in Beaugency, a region along the Loire River.[19] After the authenticity of the Beaugency case was widely reported, American physician Henry A. Martin sent an agent on his behalf to purchase samples.[20] Martin became fiercely insistent about the authenticity of his stock—he claimed he had received samples from "the 258th, 259th, and 260th animal of Dr. DePaul's series, beginning with the heifer of Beaugency."[21] By the 1880s, Martin's farm outside of Boston, Massachusetts, had vaccinated "at least five thousand animals," and provided many of the most reputable vaccine farms in the United States with their supply of the virus.[22] But the virus alone was not enough. Vaccine farm proprietors developed specific production and marketing techniques to cultivate favorable reputations.

CULTIVATION AND SANITATION

The enterprising physicians who owned and operated vaccine farms debated the finer points of vaccine cultivation, but their methods were broadly similar. To begin the process, physicians would move cows to an operating room with stanchions or strap the animals to tables. Cows were then vaccinated by lancet incisions along their bellies and buttocks.[23] This was done anywhere from 10 to 30 times on each animal (Figure 1).[24] Some vaccine producers left incisions to heal in the open air, while others protected the developing lesions with cotton and bandages. Once the cow had contracted the disease, scabbing was removed with delicate washing or scraping, and the lymph that leaked from cows' lesions was collected and poured over lancet tips, which were then left to dry. Some farms stored the liquid in pipettes, selling these tubes of lymph for a higher cost to physicians who preferred to dress their own lancet tips.[25] Regardless of their technique, vaccine farm proprietors and their customers agreed that sanitation was paramount.

The Civil War had thrown the importance of sanitation into sharp relief. In the aftermath, many American cities established boards of health. These boards were responsible for a range of interventions, including building sewers, relocating slaughterhouses, ensuring a clean water supply, and improving ventilation. At the time, public health policy was based on the idea that disease was caused by miasma, or "bad air," produced by human waste or decaying plant or animal matter.[26] Perhaps unsurprisingly, as cities grew over the course of the 19th century, illness became associated with dirty urban environments, while the countryside was seen as a healthful place where one might go to heal.[27] In fact, life in the country was thought to be so restorative that farming, while notoriously laborious, was still seen as a profession "favorable to the enjoyment of sound health."[28] Vaccination raised concerns about bodily purity, but vaccine farms provided an opportunity to associate the practice with the healing power of rural life.

Physicians keenly observed their environmental surroundings in an effort to preserve the health of their patients.[29] Those who established vaccine farms, then, thought carefully about where they should be located and communicated this decision-making process to their potential customers.

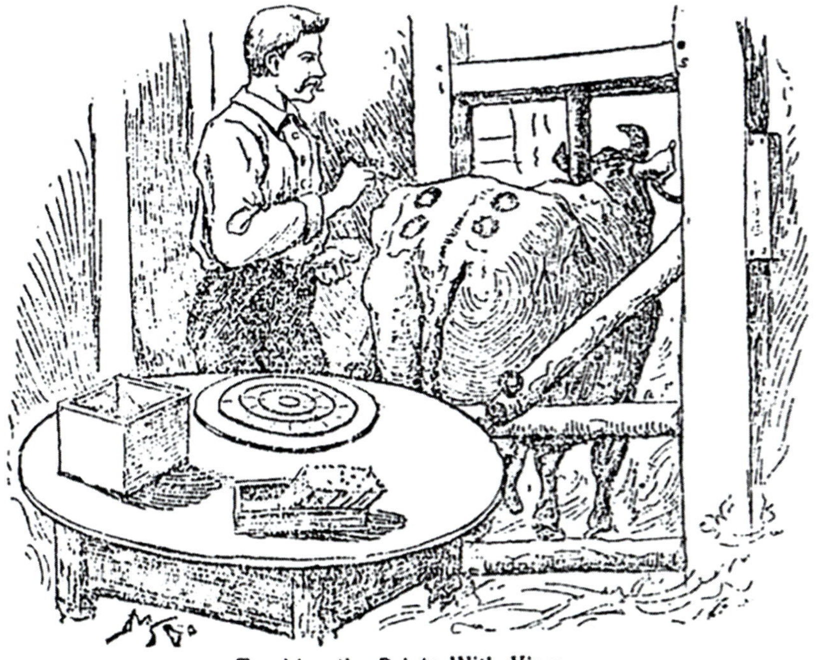

FIGURE 1— **An Artist's Rendering of the Process of Harvesting the Vaccine From an Infected Cow**

Source. "Points for Inoculation. Where Vaccine Virus Is Grown for Use Against Small-Pox," *St Louis Post-Dispatch*, July 22, 1894: 22.

AJPH February 2024, Vol. 114, No. 2

For instance, physician Hamill M. Alexander opened a vaccine farm in Marietta, Pennsylvania, which he called Lancaster County Vaccine Farms. Alexander chose Marietta because he was convinced that vaccine farms thrived in "open country, where pure air, perfect cleanliness and the best sanitary conditions," could be achieved.[30] Alexander implored his fellow vaccine farmers to keep their operations "well ventilated . . . free from filth . . . and entirely free from foul or impure air."[31] Advertisements for the Lancaster County Vaccine Farms showed a pastoral scene with green fields and rolling hills. Such images emphasized that these natural spaces were located far from the dirt and pollution of urban environments (Figure 2). Vaccine farm proprietors ascribed to the 19th century belief succinctly expressed by English social reformer Edwin Chadwick: "All smell is disease."[32]

VIRAL LINEAGES

Vaccine producers emphasized sanitation to convince customers that their product was of the highest quality. But they also borrowed a strategy from stockbreeders and aimed to establish the pedigree of their viral stock. Pedigree was a record of an animal's ancestry, which conveyed information about the traits it was likely to inherit. According to 19th century stockbreeders, "the value of any pedigree will depend upon its authenticity, completeness, and the quality . . . of the animals comprised in the ancestry."[33] Stockbreeding was not seen as an effort to artificially engineer life. On the contrary, it was often

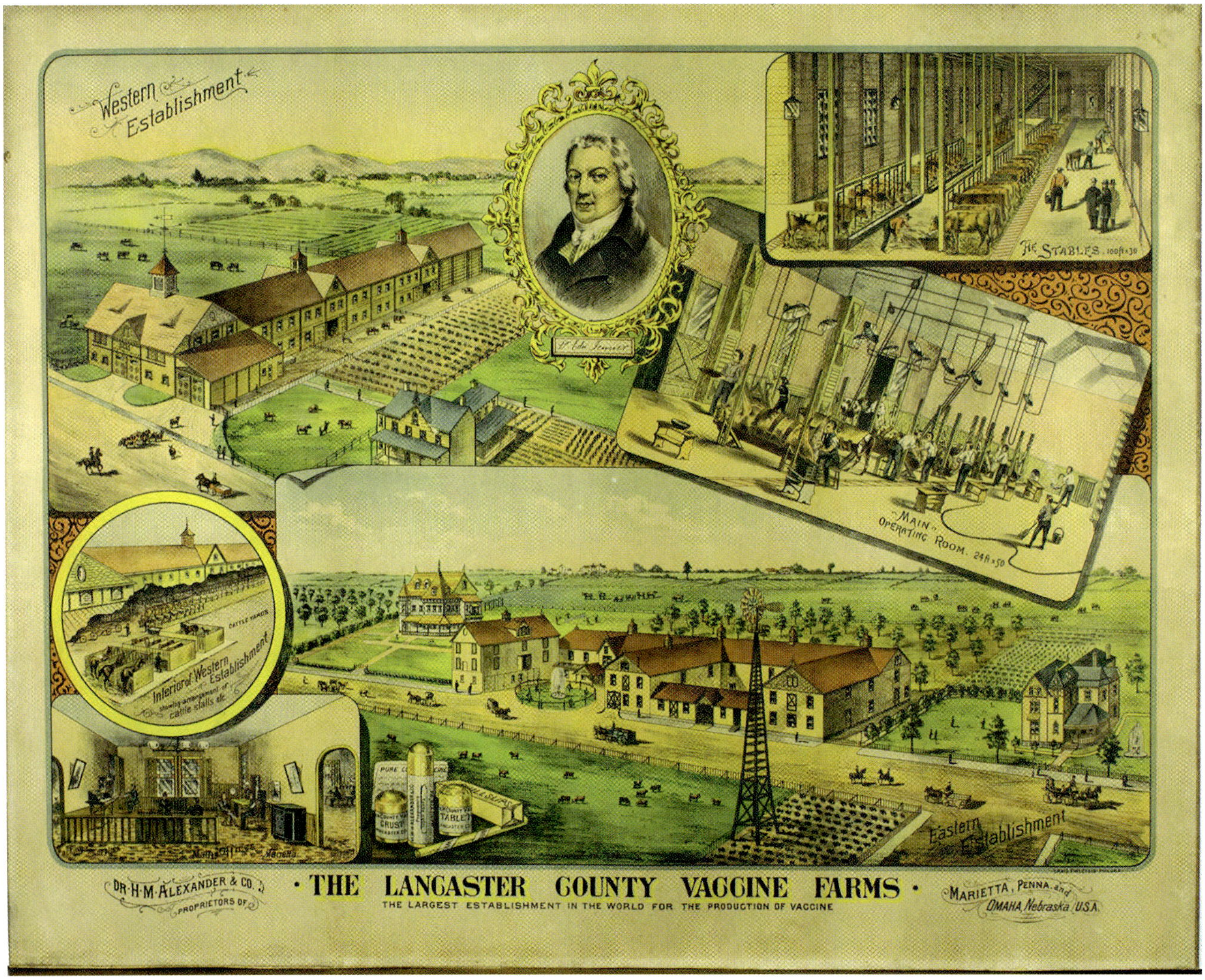

FIGURE 2— Images of the Lancaster County Vaccine Farms Emphasized the Pastoral Setting

Source. Library Company of Philadelphia, Chromolithograph promoting the Lancaster Country Vaccine Farms (Philadelphia: Craig, Finley & Co, 1885), https://commons.wikimedia.org/wiki/File:Lancaster_County_Vaccine_Farms_(17029767503).jpg perceived as a noble pursuit associated with the "dignity, social position, and breeding" of the wealthy aristocratic classes who engaged in it. According to historian Harriet Ritvo, individuals who bred cattle had to "exercise constant vigilance" to ensure "the purity of bloodlines."[34] When Martin explained precisely how far removed his viral "stock" was from the "heifer of Beaugency," he was appealing to this sensibility. For vaccine farmers, safety and efficacy depended upon carefully maintained viral lineages.

Producing Beaugency became both a point of pride and a form of marketing. The Eastern Dispensary in New York advertised lancet quills and tubes of fluid that were "the result of a continued reproduction from the famed Beaugency stock, propagated under our own immediate supervision" (Figure 3).[35] The Jenner Vaccine Farm, in Chambersburg, Pennsylvania, relied upon a famous name both for its farm and for the virus it produced. It sold Beaugency virus at a rate of $1.00 for five quills, or $2.00 for tubes of lymph.[36] The New York City health department had established its own vaccine farm, which provided for the vaccination of 50 000 to 100 000 people per year by the 1880s. The farm purportedly "propagated" virus that was "a lineal descendent of the Beaugency stock introduced into America by Dr. Martin."[37] By the 1880s, the American medical establishment was increasingly convinced that maintaining a "stock" of authenticated cowpox virus with pure lineages was crucial for maintaining the public's trust in vaccination.

This concern featured prominently in the medical literature of the time. In 1882, the journal *Medical News* launched a commission to inspect vaccine farms. Demand for vaccination was growing, the commission explained, "due to a wider appreciation of the value and safety of vaccination" and because "boards of health throughout the country" were "dispensing the virus at little or no cost." As a result, "all matters connected with its production" had become "exceedingly interesting, not only to the profession, but also to the general community."[38] The stakes of vaccine production were high. The commission insisted that anyone who discovered "an original stock of virus of the highest excellence, like the Beaugency," should ensure that it was "perpetuated by animal vaccination with almost religious care."[39] According to the commission's reports, the public had begun to refuse "humanized virus," even during smallpox epidemics. On the other hand, the public reacted to vaccination campaigns with the "freest acceptance" when municipal authorities purchased bovine virus.[40] Supply had to respond to demand.

The same strategies that vaccine producers used to maintain public trust also protected their economic interests. Martin's name became nearly synonymous with Beaugency, due in no small part to his penchant for

AJPH February 2024, Vol. 114, No. 2

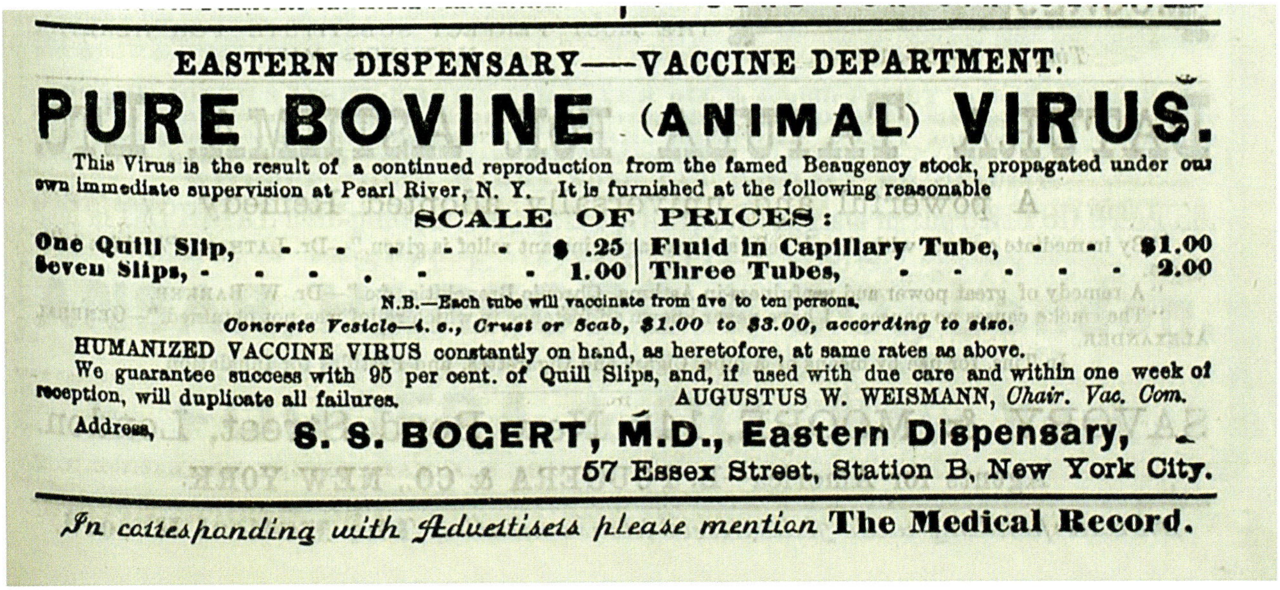

FIGURE 3— **The Eastern Dispensary Advertised That Its Vaccine Was "the result of a continued reproduction from the famed Beaugency stock."**

Source. "Advertisement 17—No Title," *Medical Record* 15, no. 12 (March 22, 1879): 27.

self-promotion. According to Martin, DePaul's original stock of Beaugency virus had been destroyed during the 1870–1871 Siege of Paris, and Martin's samples were the last to be distributed.[41] He thus positioned himself as uniquely qualified to determine which vaccine farms propagated authentic Beaugency. As in the world of stock-breeding, pedigree falsification was a serious concern for vaccine farms.[42] Martin was cutting in his critiques of vaccine farms that made fraudulent claims. "One ingenious propagator advertises that his virus was imported direct from the 'vast herds of the Duke of Beaugency,'" he complained, "doubtless a bucolic French noble, who . . . appears in history for the first time."[43] The lineage of Martin's virus, his professional reputation, and his economic success were one and the same.

By the 1880s, many physicians felt that they should consolidate exclusive control over vaccine farms. In 1883, an article in *Medical Record* warned that the Board of Health in St Louis, Missouri, had awarded a contract to a vaccine farm run by a "dry goods merchant," resulting in 10 000 vaccinations without a single "perfect success." The author argued that this was the risk of allowing vaccination to be a "purely commercial venture."[44] That same year, the Medical Society of New Jersey launched a committee to explore "Where and of Whom Reliable Vaccine Virus May be Obtained," which found that much of the vaccine lymph on the market was "impure and unreliable." One member of the committee found a specimen containing "epithelial cells, hairs . . . [and] vegetable substances of various kinds." The committee concluded that since "the propagation of animal virus" required "very exact management," the members of the society should purchase their vaccine from Martin's farm or one run by a physician with a similarly high standing.[45] These remarks foreshadowed a growing debate about regulation and inspection in a context when what it meant to be a reputable vaccine producer was changing.

VACCINE FARMS UNDER THE MICROSCOPE

The late 19th century saw the rise of bacteriology, which would transform many aspects of public health and public life.[46] Vaccine production was no exception. In 1885, G. W. McCaskey, a professor at the Fort Wayne College of Medicine, wrote to the editor of *Medical Record* asserting that it was the responsibility of vaccine farm proprietors to secure a "medical expert" who could enforce the principles of "modern science, and especially practical biology."[47] An 1896 newspaper article explained that because of "the progress of bacteriology," there was now almost no "danger of infecting a vaccinated person with the germs of any other diseases." The article went on to describe vaccine farms that used tuberculin tests for cows (killing any that tested positive), applied bichloride to disinfect vesicles, carefully ventilated operating rooms, used screens to keep out flies, disinfected knives, and had operators wear "a clean suit of white duck."[48] Vaccine producers also added glycerin to lymph to reduce its bacterial count.[49] The boundary between the farm and the laboratory was beginning to blur.

By the 1890s, boards of health increasingly relied upon bacteriological laboratories to inspect vaccine farms and the products they sold.[50] Some producers willingly submitted to inspections. For instance, in 1894, H. M Alexander suggested the formation of a "National Board of Health" with agents who would inspect "every Vaccine establishment of the country, and . . . allow no Vaccine to be sold without a registry number, guaranteeing to the druggist, the physician, and the layman that the article he buys . . . has received the sanction of the proper authorities." This, according to Alexander, was an essential step before instituting mandatory vaccination laws, and was preferable to establishing a government-controlled vaccine supply, which would undercut the "superior" lymph cultivated by private producers.[51] Alexander was protecting his own interests in a competitive marketplace. Larger and more established vaccine farms, like Alexander's, had the resources to access new bacteriological techniques and technologies.

In 1897, the Pennsylvania State Board of Health employed a bacteriologist and veterinarian to inspect vaccine farms. They noted that it was "somewhat humiliating" that three of the four farms in the state were paying little attention to "hygienic precautions or even to ordinary cleanliness." However, they found it "gratifying to our State pride" to point out that the Lancaster County Vaccine Farms operated with "the strictest observance modern surgical asepsis."[52] Alexander, it seems, supported inspections at least in part because he suspected that they would expose his competitors as subpar. Some farms incorporated inspections by or patronage from boards of health into their marketing. The Missouri Vaccine Farm, for instance, informed potential customers that its vaccine was used by boards of health in "St. Louis, Cincinnati, Nashville, Memphis, New Orleans, Kansas City, etc., etc."[53] Smaller vaccine farms generally opposed state inspections, correctly predicting that more robust regulation would make them less competitive and eventually put them out of business.[54]

FARMS BECOME PHARMA

Vaccine production, and the anxieties of those who opposed vaccination, continued to shift. By the turn of the 20th century, bacteriology had eclipsed "Beaugency" when it came to conversations about vaccine safety and authenticity. Vaccine farms gradually transformed into biologics laboratories and pharmaceutical companies, but even this was insufficient to entirely placate vaccine skeptics (Figure 4).[55] Throughout the 19th century, antivaccination leaders had argued that vaccination went against God's will.[56] In 1872, Reverend William Hume-Rothery wrote an antivaccination treatise that characterized the practice as existing "in violent opposition . . . to the Divinely-established order of nature." He went on to decry those who "would be a party to the perpetration of this unnatural deed."[57] These views persisted in the 20th century, but included added concerns about the fallibility of laboratory safety measures. Such fears were not entirely baseless. In 1901, 13 children died from tetanus in St Louis, Missouri, after being administered a contaminated supply of diphtheria antitoxin.[58] Soon after, nine more children died from tetanus in Camden, New Jersey. After a thorough investigation, state authorities could find no direct evidence that any diphtheria antitoxin from nearby producers was contaminated. But the damage had been done, and the American public viewed vaccines with renewed suspicion, even as smallpox epidemics were sweeping the country.[59]

After observing these incidents, Milton Joseph Rosenau, a scientist at the Marine-Hospital Service's Hygienic Laboratory in Washington, DC, bought samples from eight different major vaccine producers across the United States. In February 1902, he presented his findings to the New York Academy of Medicine, reporting wild variations in the level of bacterial colonies found in vaccines and what one medical journal referred to as a "ridiculous amount of

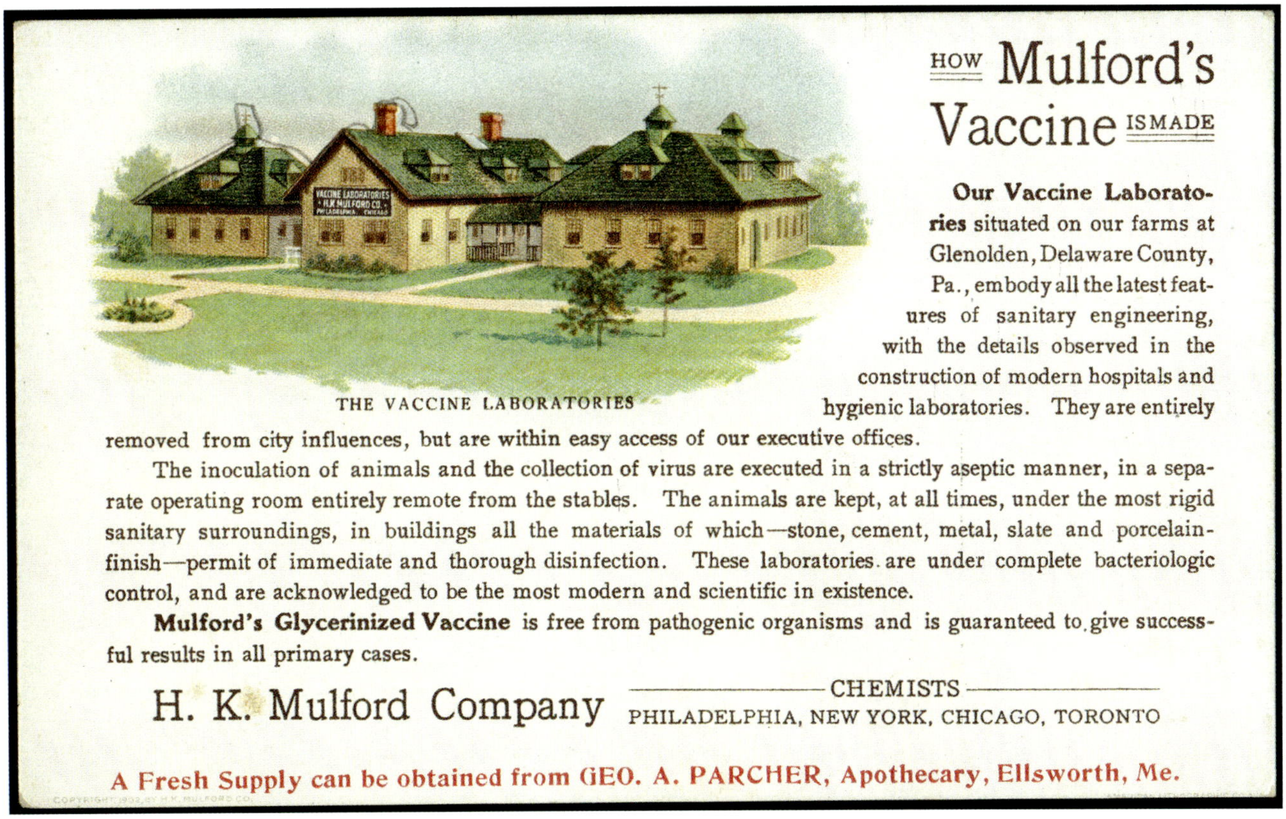

FIGURE 4— By the Turn of the Century, Advertisements Emphasized That While Vaccine Production Was "Situated" on a Farm, It Took Place in a Laboratory With Sanitary Precautions in Place

Source. Boston Public Library, Chromolithograph promoting H. K. Mulford Company (ca. 1870–1900), https://www.digitalcommonwealth.org/search/commonwealth:tm70nb293

impurity." Rosenau concluded that, "Our results so far have plainly indicated that the manufacture of vaccines is too important a subject to leave to commercial enterprise without restrictions."[60] On July 1, 1902, the Biologics Control Act was signed into law. Manufacturers of vaccines, serums, and antitoxins would need to apply for federal licensing to continue their trade and submit to inspections by a federal board.[61] This system of legal regulation markedly improved the quality of the American vaccine supply, but it also forced at least one third of biologics producers out of business. Some manufacturers could afford to achieve "a scientific image," and others could not.[62] That vaccines were a laboratory product, something that could be controlled, purified, and replicated, was considered a mark of safety that distanced them from their agricultural origins.

However, much has changed in the century since. The belief that we will eventually conquer infectious disease—prevalent in the middle of the 20th century—has faded, as has confidence that the solutions to society's most pressing problems will be crafted in a laboratory. As historian Elena Conis has shown, the most recent iteration of vaccine skepticism is buoyed by a mistrust of big corporations—particularly pharmaceutical companies—and the government. Like the earlier antivaccination movement, this one is grounded to some degree in historical reality. By the 1970s, environmental disasters, unethical medical experimentation, and medical disregard for women's health issues had all contributed to a broad loss of faith in the potential of technological innovation and in medical authority.[63] The journey of "synthetic" technologies has been similar. In the mid-20th century, many Americans thought that synthetic products were superior to "natural" ones. But when scientific innovation resulted in indiscriminate chemical use and ecological disasters, this optimism began to fade.[64]

According to anthropologist Sophia Roosth, terms like natural, organic, and traditional are now prized adjectives for foods and fibers among those who can afford them. There is a gap, then, between the way the public relates to the categories "natural" and "nature" and the ways some scientists discuss them. Synthetic biologists insist that the work they do is "undoubtedly an improvement upon nature . . . [that] life manufactured following human logic and design principles . . . surpasses and refines any naturally occurring organism."[65] This belief became even more evident as efforts to develop the COVID-19 vaccine began. In March 2020, for instance, one headline read: "Synthetic Biologists Think That They Can Develop a Better Coronavirus Vaccine Than Nature Could."[66] They may well have succeeded. But it is not clear that the American public sees it that way. While the data are still provisional, it appears that the COVID-19 pandemic did not bolster public confidence in the health care or pharmaceutical industries and may even have damaged it.[67] And, while Americans' overall confidence in childhood vaccines remains high, their skepticism about the safety of the COVID-19 vaccine appears to be much higher.[68] Overcoming vaccine hesitancy in the era of synthetic biology will require deft marketing and concerted efforts to educate the public. Scientists and those who communicate their findings to the public will have to tread carefully to ensure that when they suggest that vaccines are "better" than nature, they do not also imply that they are contrary to it. AJPH

ABOUT THE AUTHOR

Tess Lanzarotta is with the Department of History at Denison University, Granville, OH.

CORRESPONDENCE

Correspondence should be sent to Tess Lanzarotta, Fellows Hall, 100 West College St, Granville, OH 43023 (e-mail: lanzarottat@denison.edu). Reprints can be ordered at https://ajph.org by clicking the "Reprints" link.

PUBLICATION INFORMATION

Full Citation: Lanzarotta T. From farms to pharma: a "natural" history of vaccine production and vaccine skepticism. *Am J Public Health*. 2024;114(2): 193–201.

Acceptance Date: October 16, 2023.

DOI: https://doi.org/10.2105/AJPH.2023.307508

ACKNOWLEDGMENTS

The author would like to thank Catherine Mas, Alka Menon, Naomi Rogers, Adrian Young, and the anonymous reviewers for their helpful feedback on this paper. In addition, the author would like to thank Daniel Kevles for his consistent support of this project.

CONFLICTS OF INTEREST

The author reports no conflicts of interest.

ENDNOTES

1. See, for instance: Children's Health Defense, "COVID-19 Treatment and Vaccine Decisions from a Pediatric Perspective," https://childrenshealthdefense.org/ebook-sign-up/free-ebook-covid-19-treatment-and-vaccine-decisions-from-a-pediatric-perspective-evaluating-the-risks-and-benefits-for-your-child-or-adolescent-beyond-cdc-fda-or-who-proclamations (accessed October 7, 2023).
2. Melissa Suran, "Why Parents Still Hesitate to Vaccinate Their Children Against COVID-19," *JAMA* 327, no. 1 (2022): 23, https://doi.org/10.1001/jama.2021.21625.
3. See Jennifer A. Reich, "Vaccines as Unnatural Intervention," in *Calling the Shots: Why Parents Reject Vaccines* (New York, NY: New York University Press, 2018).
4. Nadja Durbach, *Bodily Matters: The Anti-Vaccination Movement in England, 1853–1907* (Durham, NC: Duke University Press, 2005), 4.
5. Sir Thomas Watson, "Smallpox and Compulsory Vaccination," *The Nineteenth Century: A Monthly Review* 3 (1878): 1006.
6. "To James Madison from James Smith, 18 June 1809," *Founders Online*, National Archives, https://founders.archives.gov/documents/Madison/03-01-02-0281 (accessed July 1, 2023).

7. George Pearson, *An Inquiry Concerning the History of the Cowpox, Principally With a View to Supersede and Extinguish the Smallpox* (London, England: J. Johnson, 1798), 67.
8. Andrea Rusnock, "Catching Cowpox: The Early Spread of Smallpox Vaccination, 1798–1810," *Bulletin of the History of Medicine* 83, no. 1 (2009): 19, https://doi.org/10.1353/bhm.0.0160. Jenner believed that he was using the cowpox virus, but recent scholarship has suggested that he may have used horsepox. See, for instance: José Esparza et al., "Equination (Inoculation of Horsepox): An Early Alternative to Vaccination (Inoculation of Cowpox) and the Potential Role of Horsepox Virus in the Origin of the Smallpox Vaccine," *Vaccine* 35 (2017): 7222–7230, https://doi.org/10.1016/j.vaccine.2017.11.003.
9. Ibid., 28–29.
10. Tess Lanzarotta and Marco A. Ramos, "Mistrust in Medicine: The Rise and Fall of America's First Vaccine Institute," *American Journal of Public Health* 108, no. 6 (2018): 741–747, https://doi.org/10.2105/AJPH.2018.304348.
11. Nadja Durbach, "'They Might as Well Brand Us': Working-Class Resistance to Compulsory Vaccination in Victorian England," *Social History of Medicine* 13, no. 1, (2000): 47, https://doi.org/10.1093/shm/13.1.45.
12. Margaret Humphreys, *Marrow of Tragedy: The Health Crisis of the American Civil War* (Baltimore, MD: The Johns Hopkins University Press, 2013), 282–283.
13. Humphreys, *Marrow of Tragedy*, 92.
14. For instance, see: "Communications. Vaccination, Its Dangers and Their Prevention," *Journal of Materia Medica* 15, no. 12 (1876): 337.
15. Humphreys, Marrow of Tragedy, 286.
16. Henry A. Martin, *On Animal Vaccination* (Boston: The Author, 1877), 15.
17. Ibid., 11.
18. On the global spread of the Beaugency virus, see: Clarissa R. Damasco, "Revisiting Jenner's Mysteries, the Role of the Beaugency Lymph in the Evolutionary Path of Ancient Smallpox Vaccines," *The Lancet Infectious Diseases* 18, no. 2 (2018): e55–e63, https://doi.org/10.1016/S1473-3099(17)30445-0, and José Esparza et al. "Early Smallpox Vaccine Manufacturing in the United States: Introduction of the 'Animal Vaccine' in 1870, Establishment of 'Vaccine Farms,' and the Beginnings of the Vaccine Industry," *Vaccine* 38 (2020): 4773–4779, https://doi.org/10.1016/j.vaccine.2020.05.037.
19. Martin, *On* Animal Vaccination, 15.
20. Ibid., 11.
21. Ibid., 17.
22. Henry A. Martin, "Anti-Vaccinism," *North American Review* 134 (1882): 375.
23. D.D. Gilbert, "The Production of Vaccine Virus," *Boston Medical and Surgical Journal*, 130, no. 18 (1894): 435.
24. "A Farm for the Production of Vaccine Virus," *Southern Planter and Farmer* 37, no. 5 (1876): 355.
25. "To Outwit a Plague: Work of the 'Vaccine Farms' in the United States," *Chicago Daily Tribune*, March 18, 1894: 41.
26. John Duffy, *The Sanitarians: A History of American Public Health* (Urbana, IL: University of Illinois Press, 1992), 119–132.
27. Susan Sontag, "Disease as Political Metaphor," *New York Review of Books*, February 23, 1978.
28. Quoted in Sheila Rothman, *Living in the Shadow of Death: Tuberculosis and the Social Experience of Illness in American History* (New York, NY: BasicBooks, 1994), 47.
29. Linda Nash, *Inescapable Ecologies: A History of Environment, Disease, and Knowledge* (Berkeley, CA: The University of California Press, 2006), 5.
30. G.M.B, "Obituary: Dr. H.M. Alexander," *The American Journal of Pharmacy* 76, no. 1 (1904): 37.
31. H.M. Alexander, "Vaccine Virus," *Medical and Surgical Reporter* 70, no. 7 (1894), 239.
32. Quoted in Stephen Halliday, "Death and Miasma in Victorian London: An Obstinate Belief," *British Medical Journal* 323, no. 7327 (2001): 1469, https://doi.org/10.1136/bmj.323.7327.1469.
33. Manly Miles, *Stock-Breeding: A Practical Treatise on the Applications of the Laws of Development and Heredity to the Improvement and Breeding of Domestic Animals* (New York, NY: D. Appleton and Co, 1878), 337–339.
34. Harriet Ritvo, *The Animal Estate: The English and Other Creatures in the Victorian Age* (Cambridge, MA: Harvard University Press, 1987), 60–61.
35. "Advertisement 19—No Title," *Medical Record* 15, no. 12 (1879): 27.
36 "Advertisement 19—No Title," *Medical Record* 19, no. 10 (1881): 13. $1.00 in 1881 amounts to approximately $30.00 in 2023.
37. "Special Article. The Medical News Commission of the Management of Vaccine Farms on the Propagation of Bovine Virus," *Medical News* 40, no. 17 (1882): 463.
38. "The Medical News Commission on Vaccine Farms," *Medical News* 40, no. 15 (1882): 411.
39. "Special Article. The Medical News Commission of the Management of Vaccine Farms on the Propagation of Bovine Virus," *Medical News* 40, no. 19 (1882): 521.
40. "Special Article. The Medical News Commission of the Management of Vaccine Farms on the Propagation of Bovine Virus," *Medical News* 40, no. 21 (1882): 579.
41. Martin, *On Animal Vaccination*, 17.
42. Ritvo, *The Animal Estate*, 61.
43. Martin, "Anti-Vaccinism," 375.
44. "Bovine Virus and Commercial Enterprise," *Medical Record* 24, no. 12 (1883): 318.
45. "Reports of Societies: Medical Society of New Jersey," *Medical Record* 23, no. 24 (1883): 655.
46. See: Nancy Tomes, *The Gospel of Germs: Men, Women, and the Microbe in American Life* (Cambridge, MA: Harvard University Press, 1998).
47. G.W. McCaskey, "Antisepsis and the Dangers of Bovine Vaccination," *Medical Record* 27, no. 13 (1885): 363.
48. "Sanitary. The Removal of the Prejudice Against Vaccination" *The Independent* 48, no. 2505 (December 3, 1896): 10.
49. Michael Willrich, *Pox: An American History* (New York, NY: The Penguin Press, 2011), 185.
50. Ibid., 188.
51. H.M. Alexander, "Vaccine Virus," *Medical and Surgical Reporter* 70, no. 7 (1894): 239.
52. Benjamin Lee, "State Medicine in Pennsylvania," *The Sanitarian* 38, no. 226 (1897): 3.
53. "Display Ad 1—No Title," *St Louis Post-Dispatch*, February 8, 1888, 1.
54. Karen L. Walloch, *The Antivaccine Heresy: Jacobson v. Massachusetts and the Troubled History of Compulsory Vaccination in the United States* (Rochester, NY: University of Rochester Press, 2015), 55.
55. For a detailed study of the trajectories of the most successful American vaccine farms, see: Esparza, "Early Smallpox Vaccine Manufacturing."
56. Jess McHugh, "The World's First Anti-Vaccination Movement Spread Fears of Half-Cow Babies," *The Washington Post*, November 14, 2021.
57. W.M. Hume-Rothery, *Vaccination and the Vaccination Laws: A Physical Curse, and a Class-Tyranny* (Manchester, England: W. Tolley, 1872), 1.
58. James Harvey Young, *Pure Food: Securing the Federal Food and Drugs Act of 1906* (Princeton, NJ: Princeton University Press, 1989), 148.
59. Willrich, Pox, 168, 190–191.
60. Ibid., 194–195.
61. Ibid., 206.
62. Jonathan Liebenau, *Medical Science and Medical Industry: The Formation of the American Pharmaceutical Industry* (Baltimore, MD: The Johns Hopkins University Press, 1987), 34–35.
63. See Elena Conis, *Vaccine Nation: America's Changing Relationship With Immunization* (Chicago, IL: University of Chicago Press, 2015).
64. Sophia Roosth, *Synthetic: How Life Got Made* (Chicago: University of Chicago Press, 2017), 19.
65. Ibid., 19–20.
66. Sharon Begley, "Synthetic Biologists Think They Can Develop a Better Coronavirus Vaccine Than Nature Could," *Scientific American*, March 9, 2020, https://www.scientificamerican.com/article/synthetic-biologists-think-they-can-develop-a-better-coronavirus-vaccine-than-nature-could/#:~:text=With%20all%20due%20respect%20to,the%20guts%20of%20a%20vaccine (accessed December 14, 2023).
67. Megan Brenan and Jeffrey M. Jones, "Image Ratings of Several U.S. Industries Tumble," *GALLUP*, September 13, 2021.
68. "Americans' Largely Positive Views of Childhood Vaccines Hold Steady," Pew Research Center, https://www.pewresearch.org/science/2023/05/16/americans-largely-positive-views-of-childhood-vaccines-hold-steady (accessed July 7, 2023).

Common Patterns of Cisgender Use in Public Health Articles and Their Implications for Gender Inclusivity Efforts, 2013–2020

Anne Esacove, PhD, MPH, MSW

See also Keuroghlian, p. 142.

Objectives. To identify how "cisgender" has been used in public health articles in recent years relative to the historical origins of the term to mark normative gender and describe systems of social power.

Methods. I analyzed 352 US-focused public health articles (2013–2020) using a summative content analysis approach. I traced cisgender use by year and compared it by sample population (cisgender-only, mixed, not cisgender).

Results. I identified 4 interlocking and mutually reinforcing patterns of cisgender use: limited and narrow use, undertheorized use, use as the default gender, and reinforcing binary categorization. These patterns largely result from the narrowing of cisgender to a demographic label.

Conclusions. Cisgender is primarily used to categorize individual research participants as not transgender rather than to reflect participants' actual identity and experiences within gendered systems of power, which undermines cisgender's potential to support gender-inclusivity efforts and deepen understandings of gender-based health disparities.

Public Health Implications. Two paths for creating more robust use of cisgender are (1) supporting gender inclusivity by clarifying and standardizing how and when the demographic category is used and (2) expanding the analytic potential of cisgender by returning to its historical origins as a framework for exposing and explaining patterns of power. (*Am J Public Health*. 2024;114(2):202–208. https://doi.org/10.2105/AJPH.2023.307441)

AJPH February 2024, Vol. 114, No. 2

It is well established that gender is correlated with health in many ways, affecting rates of disability and morbidity and access to health services.[1–5] While critically important for understanding health inequities, health research "lacks adequate tools to assess gender."[6(p2)]

Critiques of gender-related measures focus on overly broad and imprecise binary variables that make it unclear what exactly is being measured and how gender influences health outcomes; erase the experiences of transgender, nonbinary, and gender-nonconforming people; and mask intra-category variation.[6–8] Even correctives such as including "transgender" and "other" response options or operationalizing specific dimensions of gender continue to evoke complementary binaries.[6,9] As the first comprehensive review, to my knowledge, of cisgender use in public health publications, this analysis builds on and extends this area of scholarship to identify how "cisgender" has been used in public health articles in recent years relative to the historical origins of the term.

As this research will show, an increasing number of public health articles have included the term cisgender over the last decade to mark people whose sex assigned at birth aligns with their current gender identity. This increased use reflects growing understanding that gender is not always consistent with sex assigned at birth and cannot be understood through a binary. Yet, researchers at the forefront of these efforts have been doing so with little direction beyond a 2-step question asking first about sex assigned at birth and then current gender identity.[10] Inclusion of the term in public health publications mirrors a broader, if relatively niche, adoption of cisgender into mainstream lexicon. For example, its use in mainstream news and magazine reporting increased from 7 mentions in 2010 (the first noted references) to 1072 in 2020.[11] With expanded use, cisgender has increasingly come to describe individual gender identity—as represented in the most common definition of the term: "a person whose current gender identity corresponds to the sex they were assigned at birth."[12(p4)] This focus is reflected in public health articles, the vast majority of which use cisgender as a demographic category that is "not transgender."

This emphasis on individual identity narrows the radical historical origins of the term. Cisgender was originally used to mark normative gender and the privileges associated with being perceived as conforming to binary gender categories.[13,14] But, beyond a label, cisgender was originated as an analytic framework to expose and describe gendered systems of social power in an effort to denaturalize the powerful effects of gender normativity (i.e., idealized and enforced standards of femininity and masculinity) and gender binarism (i.e., assumptions and enforcement of "natural" binary oppositional categories).[14–16] The shift in emphasis from a tool for exposing systemic forces to a label for individual gender identity in opposition to transgender depoliticizes the concept and obscures the intersectional disciplinary power of gender for all people.[17–19] Scholars have also warned that individualizing cisgender creates a false mutual exclusiveness and a division between normal and other that reinforces rather than challenges cis-privilege.[14,20]

This analysis of cisgender use in 352 public health articles published between 2013 and 2020 exposes 4 interlocking and mutually reinforcing patterns associated with the narrowing of cisgender to a demographic label. Mirroring critiques of gender measures and cisgender use trends more generally, these patterns undermine cisgender's analytic potential to expose structural mechanisms of health inequities and, in turn, inform health promotion efforts.

METHODS

The unit of analysis for this study was articles identified through an Articles+ full-text search for the term "cisgender" using the following parameters—database: PubMed; discipline: public health; content type: journal article; and language: English. These parameters capture the set of journals and articles that are classified by the search engine's algorithm as public health–related even though they may speak to different readers and engage different assumptions and theoretical questions. Of the 816 articles identified in the initial search, this analysis included 352 articles with participant samples published between 2013 and 2020. These articles also report on research focusing on the United States and use the term cisgender in the body of the text (Figure A, available as a supplement to the online version of this article at https://ajph.org).

With the expectation that frequency of use and the ways the term is used would be markedly different in articles with cisgender participant samples than those without, I sorted each article into categories based on whether cisgender people are part of the study sample: (1) cisgender-only sample: articles with exclusively cisgender participants (100 articles), (2) mixed-sample: articles with samples that included both cisgender and transgender people (151 articles), and (3) miscellaneous use: articles that use cisgender in the text of the article, but cisgender people are not included in the study sample or it is unclear if the sample included cisgender people (101 articles). I used participant descriptions, inclusion criteria, and study limitation discussions to determine if a study included cisgender participants, as many articles did not explicitly label the sample as cisgender even when the term was used elsewhere in the article.

I analyzed the 352 research articles by using a summative content analysis approach that entails "identifying and quantifying certain words or content in text" and interpreting this content to understand the implications of patterns of contextual use.[21(p1283)] I used both predetermined codes (e.g., the number of times cisgender is mentioned, topical focus of the research, and keywords) and codes developed through inductive line-by-line coding.[22] Codes identified through the in-vivo process included descriptions of how participants' gender was determined and if the research focused on sexual "minority" or "majority" populations.

I tabulated the data in spreadsheets organized by publication date and document categorization, then analyzed them through a systematic review of each applicable code. Tabulations of cisgender usage included all permutations of the term (e.g., cis-woman, cis-sexism). Special attention was given to change in usage over time and differences and similarities among the categories of articles. Absolute and average frequencies of use and enumeration of 4 key areas of use (research focus, keywords, cisgender-related terms, and categorizing cisgender) are presented in the Results section.

I identified 4 key interconnected and reinforcing patterns of use across the publications through an iterative analytic process of paradigm modeling to map relationships within and across codes[22] and integrative memoing to interpret and situate the identified patterns in gender, transgender, and public health scholarship.[23]

It is important to note that the articles do not necessarily reflect how cisgender was conceptualized or categorized in the research process. This analysis, therefore, reflects only how cisgender was presented in the published reports.

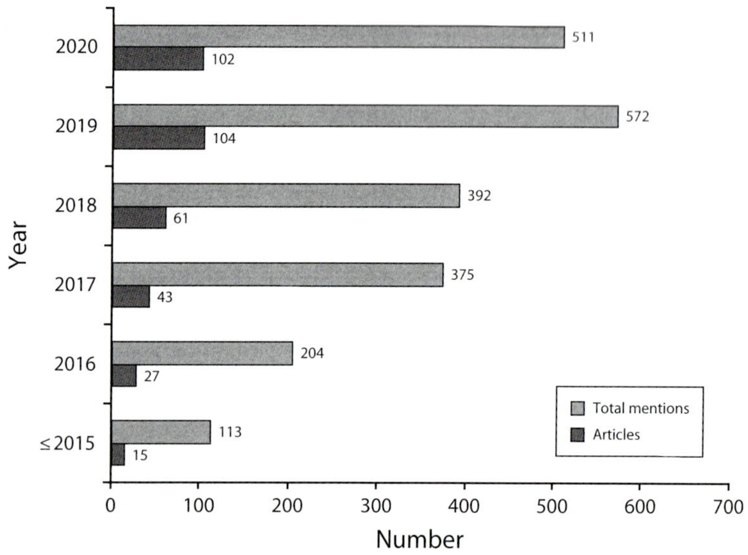

FIGURE 1— Number of Public Health Articles Using the Term Cisgender, and Number of Mentions of This Term, by Year: United States, 2013–2020

RESULTS

The number of articles using the term cisgender increased steadily between 2013 and 2019 from 15 total before 2016 to 104 articles in 2019. The number leveled off in 2020 (102 articles). There was a corresponding increase in the number of times the term cisgender or a permutation of the term was mentioned until 2019, with the absolute number of mentions decreasing slightly in 2020 (511 vs 572 in 2019). This steady increase in use over time was relatively narrow and shallow: the 816 articles that included the term identified in the initial search represented approximately 0.1% of articles cataloged in the database from the first use of the term through 2020. In addition, 36 authors represented 22% of the close to 1200 total author credits in the 352 articles (Figure 1).

Journals

The 352 articles were published in 79 journals. Of the journals using cisgender, 42% had only 1 article, 68% had 3 or fewer articles, and 6% had more than 10 articles. A third of the 352 articles were in 2 journals (*AIDS and Behavior*, 22%; *Archives of Sexual Behavior*, 9%), and 51% were in 8 journals.

Mentions by Article

Within each article, cisgender and its permutations were infrequently used. Twenty percent of cisgender-only sample articles included more than 3 mentions of cisgender; 49% included only a single mention of the term. Sixty-three percent of these articles used the term only in the methods section with the vast majority (90%) labeling the research sample and then reverting to terms such as women, men, or men who have sex with men in the rest of the article. Miscellaneous use articles (which did not include cisgender participants) were more likely to include the term more times—36% included it more than 3 times and 34% included it only once. The use of cisgender was most frequent in mixed-sample articles: 52% included the term more than 3 times, with 20% mentioning it only once. The use of the term cisgender was far less frequent than the term transgender: there were 10 207 mentions of transgender and 2554 mentions of cisgender in the full data set. This does not capture all the permutations of transgender (e.g., transwoman, transman, trans) for which there were few equivalents used for cisgender; only 8 articles included some variation of ciswoman/cisfeminine or cisman/cismasculine. Total mentions of transgender in mixed-sample articles, which are the most appropriate comparison, were close to 3 times higher than references to cisgender. The average use per article was also higher each year, between 4.5 times higher in 2016 to twice as high in 2020 (Table 1).

Research Focus

Lesbian, gay, and bisexual (LGB) people and people representing marginalized

TABLE 1— Total Number of Mentions of the Term Cisgender, by Sample Category: United States, 2013–2020

Sample Category	Sample Size, No. of Articles	1 Mention, No. (%)	2–3 Mentions, No. (%)	4–9 Mentions, No. (%)	≥10 Mentions, No. (%)
Cisgender sample	100	49 (49)	31 (31)	15 (15)	5 (5)
Mixed sample	151	31 (20)	42 (28)	42 (28)	36 (24)
Miscellaneous	101	35 (34)	30 (30)	21 (21)	15 (15)
Total	352	115 (33)	103 (29)	78 (22)	56 (16)

sexual experiences (e.g., sex work, "rough" sex) were overrepresented in study samples and the focus of articles across all years and article categories. They were the exclusive or primary focus of 71% of articles in the full data set compared with 8% with a specific focus on people who generally would be labeled as sexual "majorities." The remaining articles were evenly split between mixed majority and minority samples or foci and those that fall outside of these criteria. Cisgender-only sample articles were 3 times more likely to focus on LGB people or marginalized experiences than to have a majority focus. Two percent of mixed-sample articles had a majority focus compared with 63% with a focus on LGB people or marginalized experiences. Miscellaneous-use articles overwhelmingly focus on these groups (86% of articles), with only 3 of the 101 articles explicitly focusing on majority groups.

In addition to the focus of the articles, it was very common for cisgender to represent the "LGB" in LGBT (lesbian, gay, bisexual, and transgender) samples. This was particularly the case in HIV-related articles, which represent one third of the articles in the data set and 40% of mixed-sample articles. Most of these articles focused on men who have sex with men, often comparing them with transgender women. It was common in these articles to refer to the nontransgender sample as men who have sex with men rather than cisgender men, which reduces the number of mentions of cisgender in the article to 1 or 2.

Keywords

Of the 279 articles in the data set that included keywords, 145 included a term related to gender with a total of 186 gender-related keywords. Transgender was, by far, the most common keyword included in these articles, accounting for half of keywords overall and 70% of keywords in miscellaneous-use articles. Cisgender, on the other hand, was listed as a keyword in only 2 articles, even though 251 of the articles included cisgender participants. Even if terms such as woman, femininity, male, and masculinity are assumed to refer to cisgender people (which there is no reason to do other than assumptions of cisnormativity), these terms would represent 18% of all keywords. While transgender was included in keyword lists each year captured in the data set, cisgender was not included until 2018, 1 year after gender nonbinary[24] and gender nonconforming[25] were first used (in 2 separate articles). Only 1 mixed-sample article[26] included the term cisgender in keywords, while 30 of these articles included the keyword transgender. The keyword cisgender was included in 1 cisgender-only sample article[27] and transgender was included in 2 articles (transgender women,[28] transgender rights[29]).

Terms to Reflect Cisgender Experiences

The articles included 17 terms to reflect cisgender, representing 2 sets of binaries: (1) those that differentiate femaleness from maleness (e.g., cisgender girl vs cisgender boy; woman vs man) and (2) those that create a cisgender category distinct from transgender (cisgender, nongender minority, and nontransgender). The articles included almost 3 times as many terms for transgender, nonbinary, and gender-nonconforming identities and experiences compared with cisgender. Even when the mirror terms to those included to mark cisgender femaleness and maleness are collapsed, the articles included 46 different terms that represent gender-diverse people and experiences, including 4 terms that explicitly challenge the idea of a singular gender identity (e.g., transmasculine and nonbinary and genderqueer[30]).

Categorizing Cisgender Identity

Only 32 mixed-sample and 5 cisgender-only sample articles described the process by which participants were determined to be cisgender even though several additional mixed-sample articles included detailed descriptions of how transgender participants were identified. Only 1 article described assessing cisgender identity through self-identification, including cisgender woman and cisgender man as options in the response list for the question, "What is your current gender identity?"[31] The other 36 articles included limited descriptions of the identification process, making it difficult to determine whether these projects included cisgender as a response option or used detailed categorization processes.

Based on the information available in the articles, 3 approaches were used to determine participants' gender identity. The first was congruence between assigned sex and current gender identity. The next commonly discussed strategy was to provide a list of gender options using woman/female, man/male, and a variation of transgender or other. In these cases, "woman" and "man" without the qualifier of "transgender" were proxies for cisgender woman and cisgender man. The final method more explicitly assigned cisgender as not transgender—for example: "Persons not known to be transgender were classified as cisgender (i.e., not transgender)"[32(p2323)] and "I determined cisgender homicides by subtracting the corresponding number of transgender deaths from [public use records]."[33(p1443)]

DISCUSSION

This analysis exposes 4 interlocking and mutually reinforcing patterns present across all years and article categories that undermine the analytic potential of cisgender to identify mechanisms of gendered health inequities beyond those captured with the conventional demographic categories of woman and man: limited and narrow use, undertheorized use, use as the default gender, and reinforcing binary categorization.

The term cisgender was infrequently mentioned in public health articles overall and in the relatively small percentage of articles that included the term. This limited use was the case in absolute numbers and relative to the term transgender in both the body of articles and keyword lists. The vast overrepresentation of LGB people and sexually marginalized experiences in articles that used the term narrows the applicability of cisgender to these groups and makes it appear to be less salient for sexual "majority" people.

As a demographic identity variable, cisgender should represent a characteristic that is salient to an individual or group. The results show that the classification "cisgender" is overwhelmingly assigned to study participants, rather than assessed through self-identification; hence, it is unclear what meaning, if any, the term holds for participants. A large proportion of people for whom the label would be analytically appropriate likely are not familiar with the term or, even if they are, do not adopt cisgender as their personal identity. If the classification of cisgender is being used to represent gendered power relations that organize life chances and health status through interpersonal, institutional, political, cultural, and other systemic forces rather than a demographic category, personal gender identification is less important. Yet, most articles do not situate the research in this way. For example, only 10 of the 352 articles included analytical concepts that situate cisgender in social conditions (e.g., cisgenderism or cisnormative). As a result, it is unclear if the term represents the gender identities or experiences intended by researchers or how cisgender categories represent people or experiences that are distinct from the unqualified categories of woman and man.

People whose assigned sex and gender identity align or who self-identify as "woman" or "man" are categorized as cisgender in the articles unless they are explicitly identified as transgender. Cisgender was also the referent category to which transgender people were compared in almost every article, regardless of whether the study included cisgender participants or not. This default to cisgender is counter to the original intent of the term to disrupt the assumption of "nontransgender status" unless proven otherwise.[14,15] It also forces people to disclose transgender, nonbinary, and gender-nonconforming experiences or noncisgender identities to avoid potential erasure and misgendering, a forced visibility that is not required of people who more easily conform to the categorization of cisgender.

Another original intent of the term was to denaturalize binary classifications of gender.[16] Yet, most articles that used the term organize gender by 1 of 2 oppositional classifications. A new binary classification explicitly dichotomizes gender identity as "cisgender" or "transgender." This happened in several ways including setting up a transgender "problem" in comparison with cisgender people and comparing transgender and cisgender samples in studies. The second classification system, which is used in a quarter of mixed-sample articles, sorts participants by a reconfigured trinary gender schema: (cis)woman, (cis)man, and transgender.

Area for Future Research

This analysis included only US-focused studies to minimize variabilities of

AJPH February 2024, Vol. 114, No. 2

country-specific reporting standards and cultural conventions that configure how and when the term is used. Comparing patterns of use found in US-focused and non–US-focused studies is a potentially fruitful area of inquiry for understanding how evolving gender categories are used in public health research and for identifying ways to address the shortcomings of its current use in US-focused studies.

Public Health Implications

Increasing use of the term "cisgender" in public health research reflects growing understanding that gender is not always consistent with sex assigned at birth and cannot be understood through a binary. However, using cisgender to categorize individual research participants as not transgender, rather than to reflect participants' actual identity and experiences within gender and other systems of power, narrows the historical origins of the term and undermines cisgender's potential to deepen understandings of the pervasive structural and social intersectional systems through which gender contributes to health inequalities.

While it is understandable that cisgender is used as a demographic identifier in articles that aim to quantify health-related outcomes through gender category comparisons (e.g., women vs men; transgender vs cisgender), current patterns of this use make it unclear what specifically cisgender is meant to capture, the operational meaning of sex–gender congruence, or what understandings are gained by its use. The narrow and limited use of the label also weakens efforts to destabilize cisgender privilege by making visible that which is usually unmarked. Clarifying and standardizing how and when cisgender is used in public health publications would address limitations of the demographic label and better support gender inclusivity efforts.

Returning cisgender to its historical origins as a framework for exposing and explaining patterns of social power would go further than demographic variable reforms to address the shortcomings of current patterns of cisgender use. This reconceptualization could also address many of the critiques of gender-related variables more broadly by capturing the social and structural mechanisms through which gender operates and how these mechanisms undermine (and support) health for all people regardless of gender, understandings that could better explain patterns of health disparities and contribute to more effective health promotion efforts (see Appendix, available as a supplement to the online version of this article at https://ajph.org for specific recommendations). AJPH

ABOUT THE AUTHOR

Anne Esacove is a visiting scholar at the SexGen Lab, School of Social Policy and Practice, University of Pennsylvania, Philadelphia.

CORRESPONDENCE

Correspondence should be sent to Anne Esacove, 3701 Locust Walk, McNeil Building 518, School of Social Policy and Practice, Philadelphia, PA 19104-6214 (e-mail: esacove@upenn.edu). Reprints can be ordered at https://ajph.org by clicking the "Reprints" link.

PUBLICATION INFORMATION

Full Citation: Esacove A. Common patterns of cisgender use in public health articles and their implications for gender inclusivity efforts, 2013–2020. *Am J Public Health*. 2024;114(2): 202–208.

Acceptance Date: September 3, 2023.

DOI: https://doi.org/10.2105/AJPH.2023.307441

ACKNOWLEDGMENTS

I am grateful for the insightful and constructive suggestions of Amy Hillier, Sara Buchman, the five anonymous reviewers, and *AJPH* Associate Editor Lisa Bowleg. Librarians Sam Kirk and Frank Campbell provided important support.

CONFLICTS OF INTEREST

The author has no conflicts of interest to report.

HUMAN PARTICIPANT PROTECTION

This work did not involve human participant research.

REFERENCES

1. Hughes L, Shireman TI, Hughto J. Privately insured transgender people are at elevated risk for chronic conditions compared with cisgender counterparts: study examines risks for chronic conditions among privately insured transgender people with their cisgender counterparts. *Health Aff (Millwood)*. 2021;40(9):1440–1448. https://doi.org/10.1377/hlthaff.2021.00546
2. James SE, Herman JL, Rankin S, Keisling M, Mottet L, Anafi M. The Report of the 2015 US Transgender Survey. Washington, DC: National Center for Transgender Equality; 2016.
3. Read JG, Gorman BK. Gender and health revisited. In: Pescosolido BA, Martin JK, McLeod JD, Rogers A, eds. *Handbook of the Sociology of Health, Illness, and Healing*. Handbooks of Sociology and Social Research. New York, NY: Springer New York; 2011:411–429. https://doi.org/10.1007/978-1-4419-7261-3_21
4. Riecher-Rössler A. Sex and gender differences in mental disorders. *Lancet Psychiatry*. 2017;4(1):8–9. https://doi.org/10.1016/S2215-0366(16)30348-0
5. Rapp KS, Volpe VV, Hale TL, Quartararo DF. State-level sexism and gender disparities in health care access and quality in the United States. *J Health Soc Behav*. 2022;63(1):2–18. https://doi.org/10.1177/00221465211058153
6. Nielsen MW, Stefanick ML, Peragine D, et al. Gender-related variables for health research. *Biol Sex Differ*. 2021;12(1):23. https://doi.org/10.1186/s13293-021-00366-3
7. Lindqvist A, Sendén MG, Renström EA. What is gender, anyway: a review of the options for operationalising gender. *Psychol Sex*. 2021;12(4):332–344. https://doi.org/10.1080/19419899.2020.1729844
8. Magliozzi D, Saperstein A, Westbrook L. Scaling up: representing gender diversity in survey research. *Socius*. 2016;2:237802311666435. https://doi.org/10.1177/2378023116664352
9. Westbrook L, Saperstein A. New categories are not enough: rethinking the measurement of sex and gender in social surveys. *Gend Soc*. 2015;29(4):534–560. https://doi.org/10.1177/0891243215584758
10. GenIUSS Group. Best practices for asking questions to identify transgender and other gender minority respondents on population-based surveys. Los Angeles, CA: The Williams Institute; 2014.
11. Associated Press Online Text Archive. Gale Academic Onefile. Available at: https://go-gale-com.proxy.library.upenn.edu/ps/start.do?p=AONE&u=upenn_main. Accessed May 16, 2022.
12. Bates N, Chin M, Becker T, et al, eds. *Measuring Sex, Gender Identity, and Sexual Orientation*. Washington, DC: The National Academies Press; 2022. https://doi.org/10.17226/26424
13. Enke F. Cisgender as a term. In: *The SAGE Encyclopedia of Trans Studies*. Thousand Oaks, CA: SAGE

Publications; 2021. https://doi.org/10.4135/9781544393858.n43

14. Cava P. Cisgender and cissexual. In: Wong A, Wickramasinghe M, Hoogland R, Naples NA, eds. *The Wiley Blackwell Encyclopedia of Gender and Sexuality Studies.* Singapore: John Wiley & Sons Ltd; 2016:1–4. https://doi.org/10.1002/9781118663219.wbegss131
15. Ansara YG, Berger I. Cisgenderism. In: Wong A, Wickramasinghe M, Hoogland R, Naples NA, eds. *The Wiley Blackwell Encyclopedia of Gender and Sexuality Studies.* Singapore: John Wiley & Sons Ltd; 2016:1–3. https://doi.org/10.1002/9781118663219.wbegss426
16. Stryker S. *Transgender History: The Roots of Today's Revolution.* 2nd ed. Berkeley, CA: Seal Press; 2017.
17. Hamilton LT, Armstrong EA, Seeley JL, Armstrong EM. Hegemonic femininities and intersectional domination. *Sociol Theory.* 2019;37(4):315–341. https://doi.org/10.1177/0735275119888248
18. Hill Collins P. *Black Feminist Thought: Knowledge, Consciousness, and the Politics of Empowerment.* 30th anniversary edition. New York, NY: Routledge; 2022.
19. Butler J. *Gender Trouble: Feminism and the Subversion of Identity.* New York, NY: Routledge; 1999.
20. Henningsen K. Cisgender or cis. In: Chiang H, ed. *Global Encyclopedia of Lesbian, Gay, Bisexual, Transgender, and Queer (LGBTQ) History.* Farmington Hills, MI: Galea Cengage Company; 2019:357–363.
21. Hsieh HF, Shannon SE. Three approaches to qualitative content analysis. *Qual Health Res.* 2005;15(9):1277–1288. https://doi.org/10.1177/1049732305276687
22. Strauss AL, Corbin JM. *Basics of Qualitative Research: Grounded Theory Procedures and Techniques.* Newbury Park, CA: Sage Publications; 1990.
23. Emerson RM, Fretz RI, Shaw LL. *Writing Ethnographic Fieldnotes.* 2nd ed. Chicago, IL: The University of Chicago Press; 2011. https://doi.org/10.7208/chicago/9780226206868.001.0001
24. Stewart MK, Archie DS, Marshall SA, Allison MK, Robinson C. Transform Health Arkansas: a transgender-led partnership engaging transgender/non-binary Arkansans in defining health research priorities. *Prog Community Health Partnersh.* 2017;11(4):427–439. https://doi.org/10.1353/cpr.2017.0050
25. Chisolm-Straker M, Jardine L, Bennouna C, et al. Transgender and gender nonconforming in emergency departments: a qualitative report of patient experiences. *Transgend Health.* 2017;2(1):8–16. https://doi.org/10.1089/trgh.2016.0026
26. Galupo MP, Mitchell RC, Davis KS. Face validity ratings of sexual orientation scales by sexual minority adults: effects of sexual orientation and gender identity. *Arch Sex Behav.* 2018;47(4):1241–1250. https://doi.org/10.1007/s10508-017-1037-y
27. Todd NR, Yi J, Blevins EJ, McConnell EA, Mekawi Y, Boeh Bergmann BA. Christian and political conservatism predict opposition to sexual and gender minority rights through support for Christian hegemony. *Am J Community Psychol.* 2020;66(1-2):24–38. https://doi.org/10.1002/ajcp.12420
28. Reisner SL, Menino D, Leung K, Gamarel KE. "Unspoken agreements": perceived acceptability of couples HIV testing and counseling (CHTC) among cisgender men with transgender women partners. *AIDS Behav.* 2019;23(2):366–374. https://doi.org/10.1007/s10461-018-2198-y
29. Abed EC, Schudson ZC, Gunther OD, Beischel WJ, Van Anders SM. Sexual and gender diversity among sexual and gender/sex majorities: insights via sexual configurations theory. *Arch Sex Behav.* 2019;48(5):1423–1441. https://doi.org/10.1007/s10508-018-1340-2
30. Jackson Levin N, Kattari SK, Piellusch EK, Watson E. "We just take care of each other": navigating 'chosen family' in the context of health, illness, and the mutual provision of care amongst queer and transgender young adults. *Int J Environ Res Public Health.* 2020;17(19):7346. https://doi.org/10.3390/ijerph17197346
31. Scheer JR, Woulfe JM, Goodman LA. Psychometric validation of the identity abuse scale among LGBTQ individuals. *J Community Psychol.* 2019;47(2):371–384. https://doi.org/10.1002/jcop.22126
32. Towe VL, Wiewel EW, Zhong Y, Linnemayr S, Johnson R, Rojas J. A randomized controlled trial of a rapid re-housing intervention for homeless persons living with HIV/AIDS: impact on housing and HIV medical outcomes. *AIDS Behav.* 2019;23(9):2315–2325. https://doi.org/10.1007/s10461-019-02461-4
33. Dinno A. Homicide rates of transgender individuals in the United States: 2010–2014. *Am J Public Health.* 2017;107(9):1441–1447. https://doi.org/10.2105/AJPH.2017.303878

Regulations and Funding to Create Enterprise Architecture for a Nationwide Health Data Ecosystem

Gabriel Seidman, DrPH, Ahmad AlKasir, DrPH, MPH, MHCM, Kate Ricker, MS, J. T. Lane, MPH, Anne B. Zink, MD, and Michelle A. Williams, ScD, SM

See also Levi, p. 144.

The COVID-19 pandemic highlighted the United States' lack of a nationwide infrastructure for collecting, sharing, and using health data, especially for secondary uses (e.g., population health management and public health). The federal government is taking several important steps to upgrade the nation's health data ecosystem—notably, the Centers for Disease Control and Prevention's Data Modernization Initiative and the Office of the National Coordinator for Health Information Technology's Trusted Exchange Framework and Common Agreement.

However, substantial barriers remain. Inconsistent regulations, infrastructure, and governance across federal and state levels and between states significantly impede the exchange and analysis of health data. Siloed systems and insufficient funding block effective integration of clinical, public health, and social determinants data within and between states.

In this analytic essay, we propose strategies to develop a nationwide health data ecosystem. We focus on providing federal guidance and incentives to develop state-designated entities responsible for the collection, integration, and analysis of clinical, public health, social determinants of health, claims, administrative, and other relevant data. These recommendations include a regulatory clearinghouse, federal guidance, model legislation and templated regulation, funding to incentive enterprise architecture, regulatory sandboxes, and a 3-pronged research agenda. (*Am J Public Health*. 2024;114(2): 209–217. https://doi.org/10.2105/AJPH.2023.307477)

AJPH February 2024, Vol. 114, No. 2

COVID-19 exposed long-standing problems with the US health data infrastructure, with consequent impacts on public and population health. By mid-2021, 36 states did not publicly report COVID-19 cases, hospitalizations, and deaths regularly.[1] Despite US Department of Health and Human Services' (HHS's) 2020 guidance on collecting and reporting race and ethnicity data, the Government Accountability Office found that states and jurisdictions were missing these data for almost half of vaccine recipients, raising concerns over equitable vaccine delivery.[2,3]

The inability to rapidly collect and share meaningful data hampered the pandemic response. Public health agencies' inability to electronically receive and use data was the biggest barrier to hospitals reporting electronic surveillance data, followed by interface issues and problems extracting data from electronic health records (EHRs).[4] Recognizing these gaps, the President's COVID-19 Health Equity Task Force recommended a nationwide data ecosystem to improve public health and health equity.[5] Many government agencies, independent bodies, and networks of experts made similar recommendations[5–14] (Appendix A, available as a supplement to the online version of this article at https://www.ajph.org). Although each emphasizes different priorities and use cases, they fundamentally advocate the same thing: a nationwide health data ecosystem that can routinely and systematically collect, share, and use health data for secondary uses (i.e., uses of health data not directly at the individual patient level, including but not limited to population-level analysis, research, quality or safety measurement, and public health).[15]

Even before the pandemic, barriers to the collection and utilization of health data contributed to costly challenges. The Council of State and Territorial Epidemiologists highlights barriers to timely and broad health information exchange, with negative health consequences across multiple case studies: the opioid epidemic, infectious disease surveillance, natural disaster response, and foodborne illness surveillance.[11] Data issues contribute to the $760 to $935 billion in wasted health care spending, or roughly 25% of all health care spending in the United States.[16] (We use "health information exchange" [HIE] to refer to the act of information exchange and "health information organization" [HIO] when referring to organizations that conduct and coordinate exchange.)

This article discusses the importance of a "nationwide health data ecosystem," by which we mean a system with appropriate enterprise architecture and governance to routinely and systematically collect, integrate, and analyze clinical, public health, social determinants of health (SDOH), claims, administrative, and other relevant data. This nationwide ecosystem would retain existing authorities for state, tribal, local, and territorial (STLT) agencies to manage their health data but would have consistent architecture to allow data sharing across and between STLT jurisdictions, agencies, and the federal government. In particular, it would be supported by a single designated entity in each state (and tribal and territorial jurisdictions, as needed) with the authority and capabilities to provide a common set of core functions. This approach to a nationwide health data ecosystem is consistent with the World Health Organization's recommendation that countries develop "exchanged digital health architecture."[17] In saying "nationwide" rather than "federal," we mean an ecosystem encompassing the entire country, which requires infrastructure development, standards implementation, and leadership at the federal and STLT levels.

BENEFITS OF A NATIONWIDE HEALTH DATA ECOSYSTEM

Before assessing how to achieve a nationwide health data ecosystem supported by state-designated entities, we consider whether developing such an enterprise-wide system is justified. Based on the available information, we unequivocally believe that it is, but that further research is needed to quantify economic and health benefits.

Economic Benefits

To our knowledge, the most comprehensive analysis of the benefits of standardizing exchange of health information is the US Regulatory Impact Analysis from the Office of the National Coordinator for Health Information Technology's (ONC's) Cures Act Final Rule. It found that the benefits of improved access, exchange, and use of electronic health information for primary use cases resulting from this rule range from $1.2 to $5 billion (Appendix B, Table A, available as a supplement to the online version of this article at https://ajph.org).[18] However, to our knowledge, there is no comprehensive analysis of the economic benefits of secondary uses of health data in the United States. The European Union commissioned an impact assessment for its proposed European Health Data Space, which aims to support primary and secondary uses of data through secure data exchange.[19,20] That report estimates €5.4 billion in economic benefit over 10 years from improved secondary uses (Appendix B, Table B).[21]

Public Health Situational Awareness

Well-executed sharing of electronic health information via HIOs improves public health situational awareness. For example, in Indiana, the statewide HIO infrastructure enabled the rapid development of a COVID-19 dashboard. It collected clinical and administrative data from 117 hospitals, 18 486 medical practices, commercial laboratories, and public health departments, and a notifiable condition detector sent COVID-19 alerts to public health agencies. The COVID-19 dashboard harmonized and integrated these data to identify local outbreaks and reveal disease dynamics.[22]

Maryland's Department of Health partnered with the Chesapeake Regional Information System for Our Patients to route positive COVID-19 test results to the state's contact tracing platform. Between June and September of 2021, it pushed more than 530 000 records to the state within an hour of receipt, with 99% of those eligible for investigation having a phone number on record, facilitating rapid outbreak investigations by the state.[23]

New York City's Department of Health and Mental Hygiene and New York University developed the NYC Macroscope, a surveillance system that collected data from a large EHR network to estimate prevalence for 8 conditions, and treatment and control indicators for 3.[24] It enabled the health department to monitor the health of 1 in 6 New Yorkers, compare provider outcomes, highlight opportunities for delivering preventive services, and guide policy and programs.

Population Health Management and Care

Health systems across the country also rely on HIE for population health management for a range of diseases. Two systematic reviews identified multiple studies that demonstrate beneficial impact on patient outcomes, health care utilization, and quality of care in multiple settings.[25,26] These benefits resulted from reductions in repeat interventions or imaging, improvements detecting medication discrepancies, decreased laboratory and radiology tests per patient, and better decision-making and patient transitions. We note specific examples here.

The Veterans Health Administration system leveraged the Veterans Administration HIE and partnered with a New York's regional HIO to identify patients with COVID-19 symptoms seen or diagnosed in non–Veterans Administration hospitals and alert Veterans Health Administration clinicians to initiate follow-up care.[27,28]

One study in Louisiana found that exchange between health care delivery and public health improved HIV patients' engagement in follow-up care, HIV-related health care utilization, and disease progression indices.[29] Another study from California found that HIE between ordering physicians and laboratory staff was associated with doubling the odds of antiretroviral therapy use, decreasing racial disparities in its use, and increasing the odds of viral suppression.[30]

A nonprofit HIO working in one of the poorest counties in California served as a 1-stop information portal for county agencies working with chronically homeless populations. A care coordination platform was linked to the HIE system used by county hospitals and clinics and received data from mental health facilities, probation officers, and the county jail. This allowed social workers and case managers to coordinate care for patients experiencing health inequities, without having to search in clients' physical documents or direct outreach to another agency. This approach led to a 60% decrease in psychiatric hospitalizations and a one-third decrease in emergency department admissions.[31]

Real-World Evidence

HIE can also support real-world evidence studies. For example, during the pandemic, the VISION network, a collaboration between 7 health care systems and research centers with integrated health records across 9 states, enabled the Centers for Disease Control and Prevention (CDC) to assess the effectiveness of COVID-19 vaccines in reducing hospitalizations, intensive care unit admissions, and emergency department or urgent care visits.[32]

The Indiana Network for Patient Care created a specialized registry that extracted electronic claims and clinical data on more than 236 600 patients with traumatic brain injury, spinal cord injury, and stroke, and these data strengthened the evidence linking traumatic brain injury and ischemic stroke risk.[33]

CHALLENGES AND ROOT CAUSES

Achieving a nationwide health data ecosystem for secondary uses will need to overcome multiple challenges, which have several root causes.

Challenges

The United States has made significant progress in its health information technology infrastructure, but challenges remain to achieve a nationwide health data ecosystem with appropriate, harmonized enterprise architecture. These include the following:

- Siloed public health and health care data
- Variability in HIOs
- Patchwork digitization
- Variability in all payer claims databases (APCDs)

Siloed public health and health care data. Health care and public health systems operate in digital siloes with limited data exchange between them. Only about one third of state health agencies can conduct bidirectional data reporting and exchange as of 2016, with 65% having shared data with local health departments, 49% with clinical providers, and 32% with other states.[34] Fewer than half of local health departments receive electronic data from physician practices, and only 60% receive data from hospitals. Fewer than 60% of local health departments have implemented technology to link with EHRs, and only 20% have links to HIOs. Data sharing rates are similarly low with government partners and schools, who can serve as sources of data and sites for delivering care.[35]

As of 2019, fewer than 1 in 5 primary care physicians electronically exchanged (sent or received) electronic health information with public health authorities,[36] and a top challenge to reporting to public health is a lack of capacity for electronic exchange among hospitals and public health agencies.[37] Moreover, public health information technology systems may struggle to accommodate evolving requirements for EHR data (e.g., new data elements).

Variability in health information organizations. HIOs are designed to facilitate data sharing among multiple entities, typically within a defined geographic region. Unfortunately, as of 2019, only half of HIOs were financially viable. HIOs also provide highly variable services, with only half providing any kind of value-added services (e.g., analytics for population health or quality management). Only two thirds participate in at least 1 nationwide "network of networks" (e.g., eHealth Exchange), and planned participation rates in the Trusted Exchange Framework and Common Agreement are unclear, including because of financial and operational barriers.[38]

Patchwork digitization. Many providers have not yet fully transitioned to digital records, partly because they were not eligible for funding and assistance under the Health Information Technology for Economic and Clinical Health Act. For example, a 2022 assessment of California's health information technology landscape found that while 96% of hospitals and 79% of office-based physicians have adopted EHRs, only 32% of skilled nursing facilities and 18% of substance abuse treatment facilities have adopted exclusively electronic means to store and maintain health records.[39] As of 2021, nonelectronic methods remained the most common way to send and receive a summary of care records by nonfederal acute care hospitals, and 72% of hospitals reported challenges exchanging data across vendor platforms.[37,40] Moreover, while accountable care organization models promoted SDOH-informed care, an assessment of a national sample of 22 accountable care organizations found that they frequently lacked data required to make well-informed care decisions—namely, patient SDOH data and information about community partners to address patients' care.[41]

Variability in all payer claims databases. APCDs strengthen health data capacities and support policymaking at the state and federal levels. As of 2022, 18 states have implemented an APCD, and 32 states have not. These gaps limit analytic capabilities within these states and the ability to perform cross-state, regional, and national analyses. Heterogeneity in how data users access state APCD data and in state APCD data standards also creates barriers to cross-state or regional analyses and to the utilization of the state's APCD for broader use cases and impact.[42]

Root Causes

Inconsistent laws and regulations, and fragmented, insufficient funding both cause the challenges described previously.

Inconsistent laws and regulations. A core barrier to collecting, sharing, and using data within and among STLT agencies is the inconsistencies in laws and regulations between federal and STLT levels, and across STLT jurisdictions. These inconsistencies drive variation in jurisdictions' ability to properly use health data and unnecessary inefficiency in sharing data within states, across states, and with the federal government. States have the greatest authority to mandate and regulate data collection and sharing, and how health data are regulated by states invariably impacts how they are used.[10] Given state authority and cross-state inconsistencies, a Kafkaesque web of state regulations and rules challenges the development of a nationwide health data ecosystem.

On the one hand, certain laws and regulations can enable effective collection, integration, and utilization of health data from multiple sources. One study found that HIE increased by 18% in states with regulations that made data protection less costly, and 16% in states where legislation specifies opt-out HIE consent for patients.[43] Another study found an increased likelihood of HIE associated with 3 state-level laws: state HIO authorization, financial and nonfinancial incentives for HIE, and enforcing "opt-out" patient consent requirements.[44] Appropriate laws also facilitate data sharing among state agencies.[45]

On the other hand, fragmentation and complexity of state laws pose a burden to the collection, use, and exchange of health data. As of 2015, 40% of states did not have a law authorizing the public health authority to access HIO data, and 80% of states did not have a law requiring providers to contribute to HIO data.[43,46,47] State laws and requirements from Medicaid agencies related to HIOs face significant ambiguity and variability, such as variations in consent policies and requirements for participation.[46–49] These variations create a number of issues. For instance, some state HIE laws may reference privacy, security, or confidentiality without specifying legal requirements, causing confusion about what the law requires. In other states, a lack of mandates or weak incentives limits the total number of users exchanging data, potentially preventing states from achieving critical mass in participation.[46] The federal government (HHS) often has to rely on states voluntarily sharing their data for aggregation at the federal level.[50]

Regulatory fragmentation and inconsistencies also hamper public health use cases for personally identifiable information. For example, a total of 28 bills were enacted across 17 states on public health information and reporting in 2022.[51] The most recently published survey of state regulations found that only half of states have general use provisions and general release provisions for personally identifiable information for public health use cases.[52] This creates confusion and a reluctance to use or release data out of caution by government officials.

Well-meaning but uncoordinated efforts by states to standardize how and what health data are collected can lead to differences without meaningful distinctions across states. For example, New Jersey has written into its legislation specific terms for the collection of race, ethnicity, sexual orientation, and gender identity electronic data elements by clinical laboratories.[53] Similarly, California has written into its regulations the use of the US Core Data for Interoperability version 2.[54] By "hard-coding" data standards, states may inadvertently make it more difficult to update standards as they evolve. Certain states have restrictions on what data they share with CDC, thereby limiting analysis and interpretability.[55]

Fragmented, insufficient funding. CSTE and the Healthcare Information and Management Systems Society found that between \$7.84 billion for 5 years and \$36.7 billion for 10 years is needed to modernize public health data infrastructure.[56,57] According to CDC's Web site, as of March 2023, CDC has only reported \$500 million in Cures Act funding, \$300 million through the American Rescue Plan, and \$175 million in annual appropriation in the fiscal year 2023, although additional funding may be available through the Prepare for and Respond to Existing Viruses, Emerging New Threats (PREVENT) Pandemics Act.[58] Furthermore, these cost estimates do not necessarily include costs for enterprise-wide data sets and use cases since they focus primarily on traditional public health use cases only. Indeed, federal funding to STLT often has significant restrictions that prevent investing in a true enterprise architecture approach to health data.[59]

Recognizing these challenges, the Health Information Technology Advisory Committee made several recommendations to the ONC in 2021 on funding mechanisms for the development and maintenance of public health data systems. They specifically focus on the importance of investing in disease-agnostic infrastructure and financially sustainable HIOs that can contribute to public health goals.

POTENTIAL PATHS FORWARD

Despite the importance of ongoing federal initiatives such as Trusted Exchange Framework and Common Agreement and CDC's Data Modernization Initiative, there is an opportunity for additional efforts to directly address the 2 root causes described previously.[60,61]

Changes to legislation and financial incentives are required to establish the appropriate enterprise architecture and governance for health data at the federal and STLT levels. In particular, federal leadership, guidance, and incentives can help each state designate a single entity responsible for the collection, integration, and analysis of clinical, public health, SDOH, claims, administrative, and other relevant data. Such an approach would help each state-designated entity capitalize on the benefits of HIE described previously.

Of course, any change involving health data is politically sensitive and should be designed to preserve patient privacy and security. Therefore, patients, caregivers, and respective advocacy groups are critical constituencies to engage on the following options.

Promoting Consistency Across Jurisdictions

"Clearinghouse" for health data laws and regulations. Promoting transparency on existing regulations and governance structures, and identifying inconsistencies, could help harmonization efforts. A "clearinghouse" could show current laws, regulations, and governance at the federal and STLT levels, identifying variances and opportunities for harmonization. This clearinghouse would track progress among jurisdictions to adopt legislation, regulations, and governance that conform with, or at least do not contradict, federally recommended standards and evidence-based best practices. While the National Council of State Legislatures has searchable databases that track numerous state bills and laws, they do not compare these bills and laws or benchmark them against best practices. We propose creating a clearinghouse to regularly track and compare state health data laws and regulations against one another and to best practices. It would serve as the basis for identifying needed changes to legislation, regulation, governance, and standards at the STLT level. Such an effort could build upon previous research that effectively developed clearinghouses with point-in-time snapshots of laws at the federal and state levels.[43,46,48,49]

Federal guidance, model legislation, and templated regulation. Federal guidance, model legislation, and templated regulation could help expedite regulatory development in states and avoid unnecessary divergence. Templated guidance could also be developed where existing regulations support (or do not hinder) data exchange (e.g., the Health Insurance Portability and Accountability Act).[62]

Federal guidance, model legislation, and templated regulations should offer well-researched options for standardizing the collection, sharing, and use of health data within and between the federal government and states. It should encourage each state to designate a single entity responsible for the collection, integration, and analysis of clinical, public health, SDOH, claims, administrative, and other relevant data. This guidance and model legislation could draw on the emerging concept of a health data utility, defined as "single organization or a jointly governed cooperative of a small number of organizations, ideally operated by a not-for-profit organization with multi-stakeholder governance which, through its mission and function, seeks to meet the comprehensive health data and health data analytics needs of both the public and private sector within a state."[63(p3)] It could include, but not be limited to, the following guidance for state-designated entities: the purposes and scope of data sharing, minimum data collection and reporting requirements, permitted data uses and disclosures, governance and authorities over data, including the (types of) entities with formal authority for data sharing, privacy and security safeguards, data governance and architecture, master patient indexing approach, and strategies for integrating health data with social services data.

Of course, many STLTs have different needs based on their populations and political contexts, and they require the flexibility to structure their health data for those needs. Federal guidance and model legislation could be tiered in regulatory intensity or present various options that allow states to enact laws that are well-suited for their needs and also maximize uniformity with other state and federal laws.

Model legislation has been utilized for state public health laws and, notably, can be spearheaded by federal government agencies, such as CDC or ONC, or by nationwide organizations, such as the Association of State and Territorial Health Officials, the National Council of State Legislatures, or the National Governor's Association. One of the most noteworthy examples in public health is the Turning Point Model State Public Health Act.[64–66]

To our knowledge, at least 1 piece of model legislation has been recently developed about governance and standards for health data exchange at the state level.[67] While many components of this model legislation are relevant to our recommendations, it is critical for model legislation to be developed by a nonpartisan national body with transparent funding, mandate, and processes to ensure evidence-based recommendations.

Funding and financial incentives for enterprise architecture for health data. The Health Information Technology Advisory Committee recommends funding disease-agnostic public health data systems for states and stresses the importance of sustainable financing for HIOs.[14] We agree with these recommendations and believe that they can go further to encourage funding and incentives for an enterprise architecture across all relevant health data types via a state-designated entity. The federal government would incentivize state-designated entities to develop the capabilities set forth in federal guidance, as described previously. The federal government could create a maturity model for performance-based milestones in which state-designated entities can demonstrate capabilities to receive, aggregate, integrate, analyze, and share data, and ability to maintain appropriate data use agreements with third parties.

Promoting Innovation With Regulatory Sandboxes

Regulatory sandboxes permit time-limited pilots to test emerging technologies, services, and business models. Under a set of rules and safeguards, innovations can be tested at the edge or outside the existing regulatory frameworks. This allows for pilot testing at lower costs, reduces barriers to entry for innovators, and informs future regulatory actions.[68–70] Regulatory sandboxes would enable states to experiment with HIE innovations, value-added services, and technologies that have yet to be tested at a national level, and generate the required evidence base for state policy.

For example, the Massachusetts Digital Health Sandbox Program encompasses 10 sandboxes providing a variety of testing and validation environments for new health technologies.[71] It includes the 1up Health Digital Sandbox, which provides digital health apps to request access to medical records for more than 280 million patients via a network of 10 000 hospitals and health centers. It also includes access to more than 1.2 million synthesized patient records for testing.

Building a Body of Evidence and Business Case

To our knowledge, no comprehensive estimate of the benefits of improving the usage of health data for secondary uses in the United States exists. We recommend a 3-pronged research program be supported by government (e.g., CDC, ONC) and other funders to establish evidence in support of investing in a nationwide health data ecosystem, especially for secondary uses:

1. Retrospective analysis of previous efforts: Additional research using methods drawn from legal epidemiology and related fields is needed to study the health, economic, and systems impacts of health data regulation. This would provide more evidence-based guidance for states on how to structure their health data and HIE laws.
2. Economic modeling of projected benefits: This modeling would draw on point estimates of the benefits of standardizing the collection, sharing, and use of health data to project nationwide benefits, particularly from secondary uses.
3. Monitoring and evaluation of future efforts: As the federal and state governments take steps to improve the nation's health data infrastructure, research should formally evaluate the costs and benefits of these changes. Indeed, changes in state regulations coupled with prospective research designs could help better elucidate the impacts of certain laws and regulations.

CONCLUSION

Despite significant technological and policy advances that have improved the collection, sharing, and use of health data, the COVID-19 pandemic highlighted significant, long-standing deficiencies with our health data infrastructure, particularly for secondary-use cases. We present potential future directions, with specific emphasis on providing federal guidance and state-designated entities responsible for the collection, integration, and analysis of clinical, public health, SDOH, claims, administrative, and other relevant data. AJPH

ABOUT THE AUTHORS

Gabriel Seidman and Ahmad AlKasir are with the Ellison Institute of Technology, Los Angeles, CA. Kate Ricker is with Amelia Mayme Consulting, Denver, CO. J. T. Lane is with the Association of State and Territorial Health Officials (ASTHO), Arlington, VA. Anne Zink is with the Alaska Department of Health, Anchorage, and ASTHO. Michelle Williams is with Harvard T. H. Chan School of Public Health, Boston, MA.

CORRESPONDENCE

Correspondence should be sent to Gabriel Seidman, 12414 Exposition Blvd, Los Angeles, CA 90064 (e-mail: gseidman@eit.org). Reprints can be ordered at https://ajph.org by clicking the "Reprints" link.

PUBLICATION INFORMATION

Full Citation: Seidman G, AlKasir A, Ricker K, Lane J. T., Zink AB, Williams MA. Regulations and funding to create enterprise architecture for a nationwide health data ecosystem. *Am J Public Health*. 2024;114(2):209–217.

Acceptance Date: September 26, 2023.

DOI: https://doi.org/10.2105/AJPH.2023.307477

CONTRIBUTORS

All authors conceptualized this analytic essay and contributed to the revisions and editing. G. Seidman and A. AlKasir conducted the initial literature review and drafting.

ACKNOWLEDGMENTS

The authors would like to thank the participants at the Digital Frontiers in Public Health event, hosted by Harvard T. H. Chan School of Public Health and the Ellison Institute of Technology, whose valuable discussions helped inform this essay. The authors would like to thank Clifton Leaf and Stephanie Simon for their partnership on this essay.

CONFLICTS OF INTEREST

The authors have no conflicts of interest to disclose.

HUMAN PARTICIPANT PROTECTION

Human participants were not involved in this research.

REFERENCES

1. Porterfield J. Johns Hopkins team details lack of daily data on COVID-19 from many states. Johns Hopkins University. Available at: https://hub.jhu.edu/2021/08/17/coronavirus-daily-state-reporting. Accessed December 1, 2022.
2. Krieger N, Testa C, Hanage WP, Chen JT. US racial and ethnic data for COVID-19 cases: still missing in action. *Lancet*. 2020;396(10261):e81. https://doi.org/10.1016/S0140-6736(20)32220-0
3. US Government Accountability Office. COVID-19. Sustained federal action is crucial as pandemic enters its second year. March 31, 2021. Available at: https://www.gao.gov/products/gao-21-387. Accessed December 12, 2023.
4. Holmgren AJ, Apathy NC, Adler-Milstein J. Barriers to hospital electronic public health reporting and implications for the COVID-19 pandemic: the authors' reply. *J Am Med Inform Assoc*. 2020;27(11): 1823–1824. https://doi.org/10.1093/jamia/ocaa192
5. Presidential COVID-19 Health Equity Task Force. Final report and recommendations. Washington, DC: US Department of Health and Human Services, Office of Minority Health; 2021.
6. O'Reilly-Shah VN, Gentry KR, Van Cleve W, Kendale SM, Jabaley CS, Long DR. The COVID-19 pandemic highlights shortcomings in US health care informatics infrastructure: a call to action. *Anesth Analg*. 2020;131(2):340–344. https://doi.org/10.1213/ANE.0000000000004945
7. Morrison S, Inglesby T. Building the CDC the country needs. Center for Strategic and International Studies Commission on Strengthening America's Health Security. 2023. Available at: https://www.csis.org/analysis/building-cdc-country-needs. Accessed January 26, 2023.
8. DeSalvo K, Hughes B, Bassett M, et al. Public health COVID-19 impact assessment: lessons learned and compelling needs. *NAM Perspect*. 2021;2021. https://doi.org/10.31478/202104c
9. National Commission to Transform Public Health Data Systems. Charting a course for an equity-centered data system: recommendations from the National Commission to Transform Public Health Data Systems. 2021. Available at: https://www.rwjf.org/en/insights/our-research/2021/10/charting-a-course-for-an-equity-centered-data-system.html. Accessed December 12, 2023.
10. Daschle T, First B, Wilensky G, et al. *Positioning America's Public Health System for the Next Pandemic*. Bipartisan Policy Center. June 2021. Available at: https://bipartisanpolicy.org/download/?file=/wp-content/uploads/2021/06/Public-Health-Report_RV2.pdf. Accessed December 1, 2022.
11. Hagan CN, Holubowich EJ, Criss T. *Driving Public Health in the Fast Lane: The Urgent Need for a 21st Century Data Superhighway*. de Beaumont Foundation. 2019. Available at: https://debeaumont.org/news/2019/white-paper-driving-public-health-in-the-fast-lane. Accessed December 12, 2023.

12. US Government Accountability Office. COVID-19: pandemic lessons highlight need for public health situational awareness network. June 23, 2022. Available at: https://www.gao.gov/products/gao-22-104600. Accessed April 5, 2023.
13. Health Information Technology Advisory Committee. Final report of the Health Information Technology Advisory Committee on Public Health Data Systems. November 10, 2022. Available at: https://www.healthit.gov/sites/default/files/page/2022-11/2022-11-10_PHDS_TF_Recommendations_Report_Transmittal_Letter_508.pdf. Accessed January 17, 2022.
14. Health Information Technology Advisory Committee. Final report to the Health Information Technology Advisory Committee's Public Health Data Systems Task Force 2021. July 14, 2021. Available at: https://www.healthit.gov/sites/default/files/page/2021-08/2021-07-14_PHDS_TF_2021_HITAC%20Recommendations%20Report_Signed_508_0.pdf. Accessed April 5, 2023.
15. Safran C, Bloomrosen M, Hammond WE, et al. Toward a national framework for the secondary use of health data: an American Medical Informatics Association white paper. *J Am Med Inform Assoc.* 2007;14(1):1–9. https://doi.org/10.1197/jamia.M2273
16. Shrank WH, Rogstad TL, Parekh N. Waste in the US health care system: estimated costs and potential for savings. *JAMA.* 2019;322(15):1501–1509. https://doi.org/10.1001/jama.2019.13978
17. World Health Organization. *Digital Implementation Investment Guide (DIIG): Integrating Digital Interventions Into Health Programmes.* 2020. Available at: https://www.who.int/publications/i/item/9789240010567. Accessed April 5, 2023.
18. Office of the National Coordinator for Health Information Technology. 21st Century Cures Act: interoperability, information blocking, and the ONC Health IT Certification Program. US Department of Health and Human Services; 2020. Available at: https://www.govinfo.gov/content/pkg/FR-2020-05-01/pdf/2020-07419.pdf. Accessed April 5, 2023.
19. European Commission. Proposal for a regulation of the European Parliament on the European Health Data Space. May 3, 2022. Available at: https://eur-lex.europa.eu/resource.html?uri=cellar:dbfd8974-cb79-11ec-b6f4-01aa75ed71a1.0001.02/DOC_1&format=PDF. Accessed December 12, 2023.
20. European Commission. European Health Data Space. 2020. Available at: https://health.ec.europa.eu/ehealth-digital-health-and-care/european-health-data-space_en. Accessed December 12, 2023.
21. Directorate-General for Health and Food Safety. *Impact Assessment on the European Health Data Space.* European Commission; 2022. Available at: https://health.ec.europa.eu/publications/impact-assessment-european-health-data-space_en. Accessed April 5, 2023.
22. Dixon BE, Grannis SJ, McAndrews C, et al. Leveraging data visualization and a statewide health information exchange to support COVID-19 surveillance and response: application of public health informatics. *J Am Med Inform Assoc.* 2021;28(7):1363–1373. https://doi.org/10.1093/jamia/ocab004
23. Feldman KA, Hanks A, Williams TW, et al. A state health department and health information exchange partnership: an effective collaboration for a data-driven response for COVID-19 contact tracing in Maryland. *Sex Transm Dis.* 2023;50(8S suppl 1):S34–S40. https://doi.org/10.1097/OLQ.0000000000001702
24. Perlman SE, McVeigh KH, Thorpe LE, Jacobson L, Greene CM, Gwynn RC. Innovations in population health surveillance: using electronic health records for chronic disease surveillance. *Am J Public Health.* 2017;107(6):853–857. https://doi.org/10.2105/AJPH.2017.303813
25. Menachemi N, Rahurkar S, Harle CA, Vest JR. The benefits of health information exchange: an updated systematic review. *J Am Med Inform Assoc.* 2018;25(9):1259–1265. https://doi.org/10.1093/jamia/ocy035
26. Tarver WL, Jonnalagadda P, Rahurkar S. Evidence base for health information exchange. In: Dixon BE, ed. *Health Information Exchange.* London, England: Elsevier; 2023. https://doi.org/10.1016/B978-0-323-90802-3.00019-8
27. Sherman RL, Judon KM, Koufacos NS, et al. Utilizing a health information exchange to facilitate COVID-19 VA primary care follow-up for veterans diagnosed in the community. *JAMIA Open.* 2021;4(1):ooab020. https://doi.org/10.1093/jamiaopen/ooab020
28. Jason C. How health information exchange facilitated Covid-19 follow-up. *Integration & Interoperability News.* EHR Intelligence. March 24, 2021. Available at: https://ehrintelligence.com/news/how-health-information-exchange-facilitated-covid-19-follow-up. Accessed January 20, 2023.
29. Magnus M, Herwehe J, Gruber D, et al. Improved HIV-related outcomes associated with implementation of a novel public health information exchange. *Int J Med Inform.* 2012;81(10):e30–e38. https://doi.org/10.1016/j.ijmedinf.2012.06.005
30. Cunningham WE, Ford CL, Kinsler JJ, et al. Effects of a laboratory health information exchange intervention on antiretroviral therapy use, viral suppression, and racial/ethnic disparities. *J Acquir Immune Defic Syndr.* 2017;75(3):290–298. https://doi.org/10.1097/QAI.0000000000001385
31. Boyd-Barrett C. In Humboldt, the community works together to tackle homelessness. California Health Care Foundation. California Health Care Foundation. July 16, 2021. Available at: https://www.chcf.org/blog/humboldt-community-works-together-tackle-homelessness. Accessed December 1, 2022.
32. Thompson MG, Stenehjem E, Grannis S, et al. Effectiveness of Covid-19 vaccines in ambulatory and inpatient care settings. *N Engl J Med.* 2021;385(15):1355–1371. https://doi.org/10.1056/NEJMoa2110362
33. Rahurkar S, McFarlane TD, Wang J, et al. Leveraging health information exchange to construct a registry for traumatic brain injury, spinal cord injury and stroke in Indiana. *AMIA Annu Symp Proc.* 2018;2017:1440–1449.
34. Association of State and Territorial Health Officials. *ASTHO Profile of State and Territorial Public Health.* Vol. 4. 2017. Available at: https://www.astho.org/globalassets/pdf/profile/profile-stph-vol-4.pdf. Accessed January 20, 2023.
35. National Association of County and City Health Officials. *National Profile of Local Health Departments.* 2020. Available at: https://www.naccho.org/uploads/downloadable-resources/Programs/Public-Health-Infrastructure/NACCHO_2019_Profile_final.pdf. Accessed April 5, 2023.
36. Richwine C, Charles D, Patel V. Electronic public health reporting & recording of social & behavioral determinants of health among office-based physicians, 2019. *ONC Data Brief.* August 2022; Vol 60. Office of the National Coordinator for Health Information Technology. Available at: https://www.healthit.gov/sites/default/files/2022-08/Public_Health_Reporting_Capabilities_Among_Office-Based_Physicians.pdf. Accessed April 5, 2023.
37. Richwine C, Marshall C, Johnson C, Patel V. Challenges to public health reporting experience by non-federal acute care hospitals, 2019. *ONC Data Brief.* September 2021; Vol 56. Office of the National Coordinator for Health Information Technology. Available at: https://www.healthit.gov/sites/default/files/page/2021-09/Challenges-to-PH-Reporting.pdf. Accessed April 5, 2023.
38. Adler-Milstein J, Garg A, Zhao W, Patel V. A survey of health information exchange organizations in advance of a nationwide connectivity framework. *Health Aff (Millwood).* 2021;40(5):736–744. https://doi.org/10.1377/hlthaff.2020.01497
39. Sujansky W. An assessment of the California health information technology landscape in 2022: summary of key findings. Issue Brief. California Health Care Foundation. 2022. Available at: https://www.chcf.org/wp-content/uploads/2022/06/AssessmentHITLandscape2022SummaryKeyFindings.pdf. Accessed April 5, 2023.
40. Pylypchuk Y, Everson J. Interoperability and methods of exchange among hospitals in 2021. *ONC Data Brief.* Office of the National Coordinator for Health Information Technology. 2023. Available at: https://www.healthit.gov/sites/default/files/2023-01/DB64_Interop_and_Methods_of_Exchange_Among_Hosp.pdf. Accessed December 12, 2023.
41. Murray GF, Rodriguez HP, Lewis VA. Upstream with a small paddle: how ACOs are working against the current to meet patients' social needs. *Health Aff (Millwood).* 2020;39(2):199–206. https://doi.org/10.1377/hlthaff.2019.01266
42. McAvey K. *Realizing the Promise of All Payer Claims Databases: A Federal & State Action Plan.* Manatt Health Strategies. December 2022. Available at: https://www.manatt.com/Manatt/media/Media/PDF/White%20Papers/RWJF_Realizing-the-Promise-of-APCDs_2022-12_d.pdf. Accessed April 5, 2023.
43. Bronsoler A, Doyle J, Schmit C, Reenen JV. The role of state policy in fostering health information exchange in the United States. *NEJM Catal Innov Care Deliv* . 2023;4(1). https://doi.org/10.1056/CAT.22.0302
44. Brown-Podgorski BL, Hilts KE, Kash BA, Schmit CD, Vest JR. The association between state-level health information exchange laws and hospital participation in community health information organizations. 2018: *AMIA Annu Symp Proc.* 2018:2018:313–320313.
45. The Network for Public Health Law. Data sharing state laws: summary of state laws that facilitate data sharing among state agencies. October 22, 2019. Available at: https://www.networkforphl.org/wp-content/uploads/2019/10/Summary-of-State-Laws-that-Facilitate-Data-Sharing-Among-State-Agencies-11-7-19.pdf. Accessed April 5, 2023.
46. Schmit CD, Wetter SA, Kash BA. Falling short: how state laws can address health information exchange barriers and enablers. *J Am Med Inform Assoc.* 2018;25(6):635–644. https://doi.org/10.1093/jamia/ocx122
47. Apathy NC, Holmgren AJ. Opt-in consent policies: potential barriers to hospital health information

exchange. *Am J Manag Care.* 2020;26(1):e14–e20. https://doi.org/10.37765/ajmc.2020.42148

48. Schmit C, Sunshine G, Pepin D, Ramanathan T, Menon A, Penn M. Transitioning from paper to digital: state statutory and regulatory frameworks for health information technology. *Public Health Rep.* 2017;132(5):585–592. https://doi.org/10.1177/0033354917722994

49. Byron SC. State Medicaid policy levers related to successful health information exchange among providers. Chapel Hill, NC: University of North Carolina at Chapel Hill; 2022.

50. Office of the Chief Technology Officer. The state of data sharing at the US Department of Health and Human Services. US Department of Health and Human Services. September 2018. Available at: https://www.hhs.gov/sites/default/files/HHS_StateofDataSharing_0915.pdf. Accessed April 5, 2023.

51. National Conference of State Legislatures. State Public Health Legislation Database. October 3, 2022. Available at: https://www.ncsl.org/health/state-public-health-legislation-database. Accessed January 24, 2023.

52. Begley EB, Ware JM, Hexem SA, et al. Personally identifiable information in state laws: use, release, and collaboration at health departments. *Am J Public Health.* 2017;107(8):1272–1276. https://doi.org/10.2105/AJPH.2017.303862

53. Conway H Jr, Pinkin NJ, Jimenez AM, Reynolds-Jackson V. New Jersey Assembly Bill 4253, 219th Legislature (2020). Available at: https://legiscan.com/NJ/text/A4253/2020. Accessed April 5, 2023.

54. California Health and Human Services. Data elements to be exchanged. Data exchange framework data sharing agreement and policies & procedures. 1st ed. Available at: https://www.chhs.ca.gov/data-exchange-framework/2022. Accessed April 5, 2023.

55. Centers for Disease Control and Prevention. Data definitions for COVID-19 vaccinations in the United States. Available at: https://www.cdc.gov/coronavirus/2019-ncov/vaccines/reporting-vaccinations.html. Accessed January 25, 2023.

56. Council of State and Territorial Epidemiologists. Modernize public health data: a call to Congress. 2022. Available at: https://cdn.ymaws.com/www.cste.org/resource/resmgr/data_health/DMI_Costs_One_Pager_FINAL_08.pdf. Accessed April 5, 2023.

57. Healthcare Information and Management Systems Society. Public health information and technology infrastructure modernization funding report. 2022. Available at: https://www.himss.org/sites/hde/files/media/file/2022/04/29/pubpolicydatamodernization_final.pdf. Accessed April 5, 2023.

58. Centers for Disease Control and Prevention. Data Modernization Initiative: Why sustainable funding matters. Available at: https://www.cdc.gov/surveillance/surveillance-data-strategies/dmi-investments.html. Accessed April 5, 2023.

59. Block L, Ricker-Kiefert K. Closing the gap in California's health data exchange: necessary investments and funding opportunities. California Health Care Foundation. June 2022. Available at: https://www.chcf.org/wp-content/uploads/2022/06/ClosingGapCAsDataExchangeNecessaryInvestments.pdf. Accessed April 5, 2023.

60. Office of the National Coordinator for Health Information Technology. Trusted Exchange Framework and Common Agreement (TEFCA). Available at: https://www.healthit.gov/topic/interoperability/policy/trusted-exchange-framework-and-common-agreement-tefca. Accessed December 1, 2022.

61. Centers for Disease Control and Prevention. What is the Data Modernization Initiative? Available at: https://www.cdc.gov/surveillance/projects/dmi-initiative/index.html. Accessed December 1, 2022.

62. Mello MM, Adler-Milstein J, Ding KL, Savage L. Legal barriers to the growth of health information exchange—boulders or pebbles? *Milbank Q.* 2018;96(1):110–143. https://doi.org/10.1111/1468-0009.12313

63. Consortium for State and Regional Interoperability. Consortium for State and Regional Interoperability health data utility maturity model. April 18, 2023. Available at: https://thecsri.org/news/consortium-for-state-and-regional-interoperability-health-data-utility-maturity-model. Accessed April 5, 2023.

64. Hodge JG Jr, Gostin LO, Gebbie K, Erickson DL. Transforming public health law: the Turning Point Model State Public Health Act. *J Law Med Ethics.* 2006;34(1):77–84. https://doi.org/10.1111/j.1748-720X.2006.00010.x

65. Foley M. The Turning Point Model State Public Health Act—emergency public health law versus civil liberties. *Virtual Mentor.* 2010;12(9):735–738. https://doi.org/10.1001/virtualmentor.2010.12.9.pfor2-1009

66. Khaldun JS. In context—The Turning Point Model State Public Health Act. *Virtual Mentor.* 2010;12(9):731–734. https://doi.org/10.1001/virtualmentor.2010.12.9.pfor1-1009

67. American Legislative Exchange Council. Statewide Health Data Utility Act. Available at: https://alec.org/model-policy/statewide-health-data-utility-act/2022. Accessed April 5, 2023.

68. Jenik I. Briefing on regulatory sandboxes. United Nations Secretary-General's Special Advocate for Inclusive Finance for Development. 2017. Available at: https://www.unsgsa.org/sites/default/files/resources-files/2020-09/Fintech_Briefing_Paper_Regulatory_Sandboxes.pdf. Accessed April 5, 2023.

69. Gleason P. Regulatory sandboxes give states an edge attracting innovation and investment. *Forbes.* December 31, 2021. Available at: https://www.forbes.com/sites/patrickgleason/2021/12/31/regulatory-sandboxes-give-states-an-edge-attracting-innovation-and-investment/?sh=6fe35e07003f. Accessed February 2, 2023.

70. Levin RB, Neuman BS, Kelly JM. Hardly child's play: North Carolina joins the growing number of states with a FinTech regulatory sandbox. *The National Law Review.* October 19, 2021;13(38). Available at: https://www.natlawreview.com/article/hardly-child-s-play-north-carolina-joins-growing-number-states-fintech-regulatory. Accessed February 2, 2023.

71. Martin D. Digital Health Sandbox Network. Mass Digital Health. Available at: https://massdigitalhealth.org/sandbox-network. Accessed January 25, 2023.

Use of Telehealth Information for Early Detection: Insights From the COVID-19 Pandemic

Steven Haenchen, MPH, Bridget McCabe, MD, MPH, Wendy J. Mack, PhD, Jason N. Doctor, PhD, Jeffrey A. Linder, MD, MPH, Stephen D. Persell, MD, MPH, Jason Tibbels, MD, and Daniella Meeker, PhD

See also Chowell and Lawson, p. 146.

Objectives. To examine whether the addition of telehealth data to existing surveillance infrastructure can improve forecasts of cases and mortality.

Methods. In this observational study, we compared accuracy of 14-day forecasts using real-time data available to the National Syndromic Surveillance Program (standard forecasts) to forecasts that also included telehealth information (telehealth forecasts). The study was performed in a national telehealth service provider in 2020 serving 50 US states and the District of Columbia.

Results. Among 10.5 million telemedicine encounters, 169 672 probable COVID-19 cases were diagnosed by 5050 clinicians, with a rate between 0.79 and 47.8 probable cases per 100 000 encounters per day (mean = 8.37; SD = 10.75). Publicly reported case counts ranged from 0.5 to 237 916 (mean: 53 913; SD = 47 466) and 0 to 2328 deaths (mean = 1035; SD = 550) per day. Telehealth-based forecasts improved 14-day case forecasting accuracy by 1.8 percentage points to 30.9% (P = .06) and mortality forecasting by 6.4 percentage points to 26.9% (P < .048).

Conclusions. Modest improvements in forecasting can be gained from adding telehealth data to syndromic surveillance infrastructure. (*Am J Public Health*. 2024;114(2):218–225. https://doi.org/10.2105/AJPH.2023.307499)

AJPH February 2024, Vol. 114, No. 2

The COVID-19 pandemic tested the public health infrastructure, with unprecedented public and private efforts to compile meaningful information to inform decision-making. Early in the pandemic, the Centers for Disease Control and Prevention (CDC) and National Syndromic Surveillance Program (NSSP) renewed contracts to aggregate information from health care and public health sources.[1] Further modernizing public health infrastructure is a pillar of the $500 million allocation to the CDC from the Coronavirus Aid, Relief, and Economic Security (CARES) Act. In addition, CDC launched the COVID-19 Forecast Hub, an open partnership evaluating different forecasting models.[2] While a number of improvements are contemplated for CDC surveillance systems, from monitoring retail purchases to wastewater testing,[3] health system data remain the backbone of the NSSP's real-time surveillance system, and COVID-19 efforts have both tested and reinforced the need for early arriving information. These advancements present COVID-19 as a useful test case for evaluating novel real-time information sources for syndromic surveillance, including telehealth.

NSSP collects near-real-time coded data produced during health care encounters. Data are transmitted from commercial laboratories, urgent care, and emergency departments. Automated transmissions from more than 6200 sources in 50 states deliver diagnosis codes and other information generated during health care encounters within 24 hours. CDC estimates that 71% of emergency department visits contribute to the NSSP.[4] This type of automated reporting based on coded data are efficient, particularly when codes are aligned with billing and payment requirements.[5] Early in the COVID-19 pandemic, billing codes were defined for test-confirmed cases, but the United States did not adopt billing codes for clinical or probable definitions for

COVID-19–like illness. This may have limited information delivered via NSSP real-time systems until testing and billing codes were more widely available.[6]

Telehealth-based surveillance is among a number of possible sources of leading indicators that have been proposed as information sources that might augment facility-based sources contributing to NSSP. While the diagnostic gold standard is laboratory tests, laboratory testing is not always as timely as other sources and, in the case of COVID-19, was not widely available early in the pandemic. Symptom monitoring may more quickly inform understanding of community spread and help inform planning and resource allocation.[7,8] Proposed augmentations include Internet search results,[9,10] voluntary self-report of symptoms trackers,[11] and retail pharmacy purchases.[12,13] Like these early arriving information sources, telehealth encounters do not provide confirmed test results but generate information soon after individuals' symptoms engender concern. However, unlike these sources, telehealth-based assessments can be adjudicated by clinicians with appropriate training on case definitions and situational awareness. Council of State and Territorial Epidemiologists (CSTE) case definitions are developed with uncertainty in mind—definitions for "probable" cases frequently use symptom-based criteria when laboratory tests are not available.[14] In circumstances when test availability is limited, as was the case early in the COVID-19 pandemic, clinicians' symptom-based assessments are often the best available option, but in-person examinations may present risks. Meanwhile, shifts in utilization patterns attended the COVID-19 pandemic, including relative increases in adoption of telehealth compared with other NSSP settings.[15] Furthermore, as more than half the US dedicated telehealth market is served by 4 providers,[16] adding a single dedicated telehealth provider yields broad national coverage in comparison with adding an additional facility-based data source.

With this in mind, the value of including real-time telehealth information requires investigation given the expense of adding new data sources and uncertain accuracy of symptom-based definitions.[17] In the case of respiratory infections, urgent care telehealth service providers treat more cases of respiratory symptoms than traditional primary care.[18,19] Several local jurisdictions have incorporated probable case report forms from dedicated telehealth service providers. Whether telehealth can contribute in a meaningful way to future syndromic surveillance strategy depends on the predictive value of forecasts incorporating telehealth data. Because of its large geographic coverage and relative technical simplicity, using near-real-time information from dedicated telehealth service providers to supplement existing facility-based data is promising from an information economics standpoint. For these reasons, we sought to examine whether the addition of telehealth data to existing surveillance infrastructure can improve forecasts of cases and mortality.

METHODS

This observational study compared the accuracy of 14-day forecasts using the type of real-time data available to NSSP (standard forecasts) to forecasts that also included telehealth information (telehealth forecasts; Figure 1). To minimize confounding performance factors, standard forecasts used a minimalistic approach similar to reference models in previous work[20] but did not include any outside information about demographics, policies, subnational geographic detail, or immunity. Thus, the accuracy of results cannot be compared with more complex approaches reported elsewhere.[21] The original data submitted by health care providers to NSSP was not available for comparison; public data on test-confirmed cases curated by CDC contractors is representative of (or better than) real-time information available through NSSP,[22] allowing for a conservative performance comparison between telehealth models and standard models. We also considered forecasts of deaths attributed to COVID-19 as an alternative measure given that previous work concluded that mortality forecasting has been found to be more reliable than case forecasting.[23] De-identified probable COVID-19 case rate data, based on clinical symptoms and epidemiological linkage, aggregated at a national level, was provided by Teladoc Health to generate telehealth forecasts. Taken together, these methods present a conservative perspective on the added value of telehealth information when comparing forecast performance. Statistical analysis was performed in November 2021.

The study was performed in a large, dedicated telehealth service provider in 2020. During 2020, 10.5 million encounters occurred with patients from 50 states and the District of Columbia, with 1.2 million encounters being diagnosed with acute respiratory illness or COVID-19 (Table 1). Data were aggregated and compared with the Johns Hopkins University Center for Systems Science and Engineering (CSSE) including tests, test-confirmed cases, and deaths.[22,24]

Telehealth visits were included in the aggregated data if the patient's

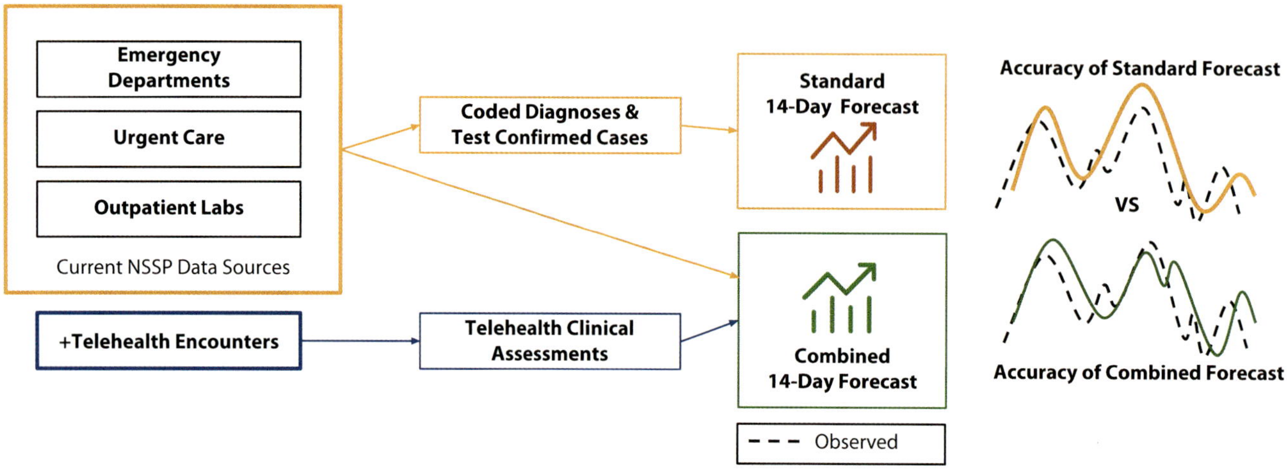

FIGURE 1— **Study Design, Comparison Between Accuracy of Standard Forecasts Using Historical Test-Confirmed Cases (or Deaths) Versus Adding Telehealth Data to Test-Confirmed Cases to Generate Telehealth Forecasts**

preferred pharmacy (used as a proxy for their current location) was located in the states included in the CSSE database. The public data include daily counts of deaths, positive and negative tests, and test-confirmed cases, but do not include telehealth-based cases.

Data Collection and Probable Case Classification

Data were collected from publicly available sources online associated with reputable health organizations, health research centers, national organizations, research journals, and academic institutions. COVID-19 case counts were taken from the different data sources, including the COVID-19 Dashboard by the CSSE at Johns Hopkins University (publicly available at https://systems.jhu.edu) and Teladoc Health vendor. Some data cannot be shared publicly because they are owned by a third party and authors do not have permission to share the data. Data may be available upon request and completion of necessary agreements.

The CSSE COVID-19 data set mortality, test, and case data collection and curation process is described in Badr et al.[22] The telehealth case definition followed the CSTE criteria for "probable case" classification for COVID-19 in the absence of testing requiring the case to meet clinical criteria and be epidemiologically linked.[17,25] To maximize consistency of documentation, in March of 2020, Teladoc introduced trainings and began collecting structured data in their electronic health record system using a mandatory screening tool documenting symptom and exposure information consistent with CSTE definitions. Screening tools and physician

TABLE 1— **Summary of Telehealth Encounters: United States, 2020**

	2020 ARI/COVID-19 Encounters,[a] No. (%)	2020 Presumptive COVID-19 Cases,[b] No. (%)
Encounters	1 200 406	169 672
Clinicians	5 050	5 050
Patient age group, y		
0–17	96 032 (8)	3 393 (2)
18–64	1 080 365 (90)	162 885 (96)
≥ 65	24 008 (2)	3 393 (2)
Male patients	468 158 (39)	79 746 (47)
Patient region		
Northeast	132 045 (11)	25 451 (15)
South	624 211 (52)	76 352 (45)
West	240 081 (20)	44 115 (26)
Midwest	192 065 (16)	25 451 (15)

Note. ARI = acute respiratory infection.
[a]Telehealth encounters include diagnosis for ARIs, COVID-19, or presumptive COVID-19.
[b]Telehealth encounters that were coded by clinicians as presumptive cases based on most recent Centers for Disease Control and Prevention guidance (see Appendix A, available as a supplement to the online version of this article at https://ajph.org, for details of guidance).

diagnostic guidance were updated as CSTE diagnostic criteria evolved. For example, when gastrointestinal symptoms were added to probable case criteria, the screening tools and guidance were updated. (See Appendix A, available as a supplement to the online version of this article at https://ajph.org, for detailed criteria and links to versions of CTSE probable case criteria.)

Outcomes and Study Variables

Primary outcomes were accuracy of 14-day forecasts of COVID-19 cases and mortality, comparing the accuracy of standard forecasts—based on a standard model using only recent history of publicly reported data—to telehealth forecasts that add unreported telehealth information to the standard model. Accuracy was measured as the mean absolute percentage error of each forecast.

Study variables include proportion of all encounters that are probable COVID-19 cases during Teladoc telehealth visits and public data on confirmed positive COVID-19 cases, deaths attributed to COVID-19, and testing rates.

Data Processing

All data were smoothed with 7-day trailing averages, taking mean incidence values over the last 7 days. Trailing averages ensured forecasts for each date were based solely on past data and not subject to day-of-week variations in case reporting. Telehealth data on probable COVID-19 diagnoses were captured in the Teladoc Electronic Medical Record, smoothed, and aggregated at the national level when provided for analysis. Aggregate overall monthly telehealth visit volumes in each state were made available to reweight public data by state. Using this information, trailing averages of daily US mortality, testing, and case counts were calculated to produce final study variables used for modeling, with counts of public data from each state reweighted proportionally to monthly telehealth visit volume.

Statistical Analysis

Means, standard deviations, and ranges of study variables are reported.

Model specification and estimation for standard and telehealth models. Forecast accuracy reflects how predictions based on past data would have performed had they been available for planning as the pandemic evolved. This is more conservative than an approach that reports accuracy of predictions based on in-sample data, and more meaningful for assessing information value in the surveillance context. Similar to other reference models used in COVID-19 forecasting efforts, our standard models do not include external information regarding policies, transmission, or other factors, with the first 14-day forecast estimated the last week in April using retrospective case or mortality data 74 to 14 days before the data used to assess forecast accuracy.[26] Forecasting was based on a simple second-order auto-regressive integrated moving average model with parameters as follows[27]: The standard models for forecasting cases and mortality include 2 days of lagged case or mortality data, a single differencing term, and a drift parameter. Model parameters used for forecasts were dynamically estimated using 60-day rolling windows throughout the pandemic. In other words, model parameters were updated daily using data available 74–14 days in advance of the date forecast accuracy was assessed. Because only nationally aggregated telehealth case rates were available, models do not adjust for demographic or geographic patterns. To assess whether telehealth adds meaningful information as a leading indicator of future events, the telehealth models added 2 additional leading indicators to the standard model as lagged regressors: telehealth-based probable cases 14 and 28 days before the target date for each forecast. If addition of these leading indicators improved forecasting accuracy compared with standard forecasts, we would conclude that telehealth may add meaningful information.

Accuracy assessments. We report the accuracy of standard and telehealth forecasts using absolute error and mean absolute percentage error (MAPE):

$$(1) \qquad MAPE = \frac{1}{n}\sum_{t=1}^{n}\left|\frac{A_t - F_t}{A_t}\right|$$

where n is the number of days when a forecast of cases or deaths was made, A_t is the mean of publicly reported cases or deaths on day t, and F_t is the forecasted value using the model. We compared the model using telehealth data and public data to the standard model that only includes public data using Diebold–Mariano tests.[28] We completed analyses with R (version 3.6.0; R Core Team, Vienna, Austria; and *tseries, forecast, lmtest,* and *MLmetrics* packages).

RESULTS

While public data do not include details of age and gender, among probable cases in telemedicine patients, the average patient age was 37.5 years (SD = 14.5); 61% were female. Table 1 shows the population was largely skewed toward working-age adults with an underrepresentation of children and persons aged 65 years and older. While all 50 states and the District of Columbia were represented in these encounters, they were somewhat skewed to populations in the South and Midwest compared with overall US population (South: 49% vs 39% in the United States overall; Midwest: 26% vs 21%; Northeast: 12% vs 17%; West: 13% vs 24%).[29] We smoothed data from Badr et al.[22] with 7-day trailing averages for model estimation. Between January 27, 2020, and December 31, 2020, on average, there were 53 913.1 test-confirmed COVID-19 cases per day (SD = 47 466.6), 1035.4 deaths (SD = 550.7), and 73 839.0 tests (SD = 50 3234.8). Over the same period, we observed 8.37 clinical diagnoses per 100 000 encounters per day in the telehealth data.

Figure 2a shows observed values of test-confirmed cases or deaths (dashed black lines) with 14-day forecasts with and without telehealth information (green and orange lines), respectively, against the background of telehealth cases (white fill). Overall, telehealth-based diagnoses rise and peak before test-confirmed cases and deaths in each wave, though relative error magnitude varies over time.

Figure 2b demonstrates observed values of deaths (dashed black lines) with 14-day forecasts with and without telehealth information (green and orange lines), respectively, against the background of telehealth cases (white fill).

Figure 2a and 2b display and quantify the accuracy of forecasting results of case and mortality forecasts using MAPE. Standard forecasts predicted COVID-19 cases and mortality with MAPEs of 32.7% and 33.3%, respectively. Telehealth forecasts improved case prediction accuracy by 1.8 percentage points to 30.9% ($P = .06$) and mortality prediction by 6.4 percentage points to 26.9% ($P < .05$). Over the entire time period, 14-day standard and telehealth forecasts tended to overestimate daily cases by 6135.6 (SD = 22 014.7) and 5846.9 (SD = 21 548.9), respectively, and overestimate daily deaths by 82.8 (SD = 327.9) and 79.5 (SD = 327.9), respectively. Directionality of errors varied over time.

DISCUSSION

Syndromic surveillance systems provide early detection and awareness of novel disease and outbreaks, producing provisional data that can inform planning and policymaking. Currently, the NSSP relies largely on information generated during health care operations: near-real-time coded data from electronic medical records and national commercial laboratories. Our results show that telehealth diagnoses based on CSTE criteria for "probable case" reporting can serve as a leading indicator forecasting death and, to a lesser extent, forecasting test-confirmed cases. This difference is consistent with previous work comparing case and death forecasts,[23] as mortality information may be less sensitive to variations in test availability.[30] We show that even this coarse telehealth data from a single telehealth service provider significantly improved predictions of future mortality attributed to COVID-19. This added value did not reach statistical significance thresholds when predicting cases, at least at the national level of aggregation used in this analysis. More complete information, such as demographic, geographic, transmission, and immunity estimates as well as information from additional service providers may help resolve outstanding questions regarding whether telehealth data independently add value to case predictions.

In light of these results, as syndromic surveillance infrastructure is modernized, near-real-time data from dedicated telehealth service providers should be considered. Reports from telehealth may give early indication of changes in epidemiology before test results are available and can provide data if testing is unavailable and only clinical diagnoses are available. Telehealth data sources collected in a standardized manner may fill a growing gap in the existing surveillance information network as in-person urgent care is substituted with telehealth and patients are reluctant to risk exposure at in-person settings.

An additional consideration is the cost and benefit of adding information inputs to the national surveillance infrastructure. The vast majority of health systems contributing to the NSSP each add only limited geographic coverage. Because large, dedicated telehealth service providers use a common information system, the cost of adding near-real-time data is comparatively low given the scope and added value—patients from all 50 states are represented in the single data source used in this study.

The common platform used by the telehealth provider we studied also allowed for rapid dissemination and updating of CSTE definitions to clinicians: daily monitoring of newly available public health information by lead physicians and medical officers resulted in timely e-mail distribution of standardized updated clinical

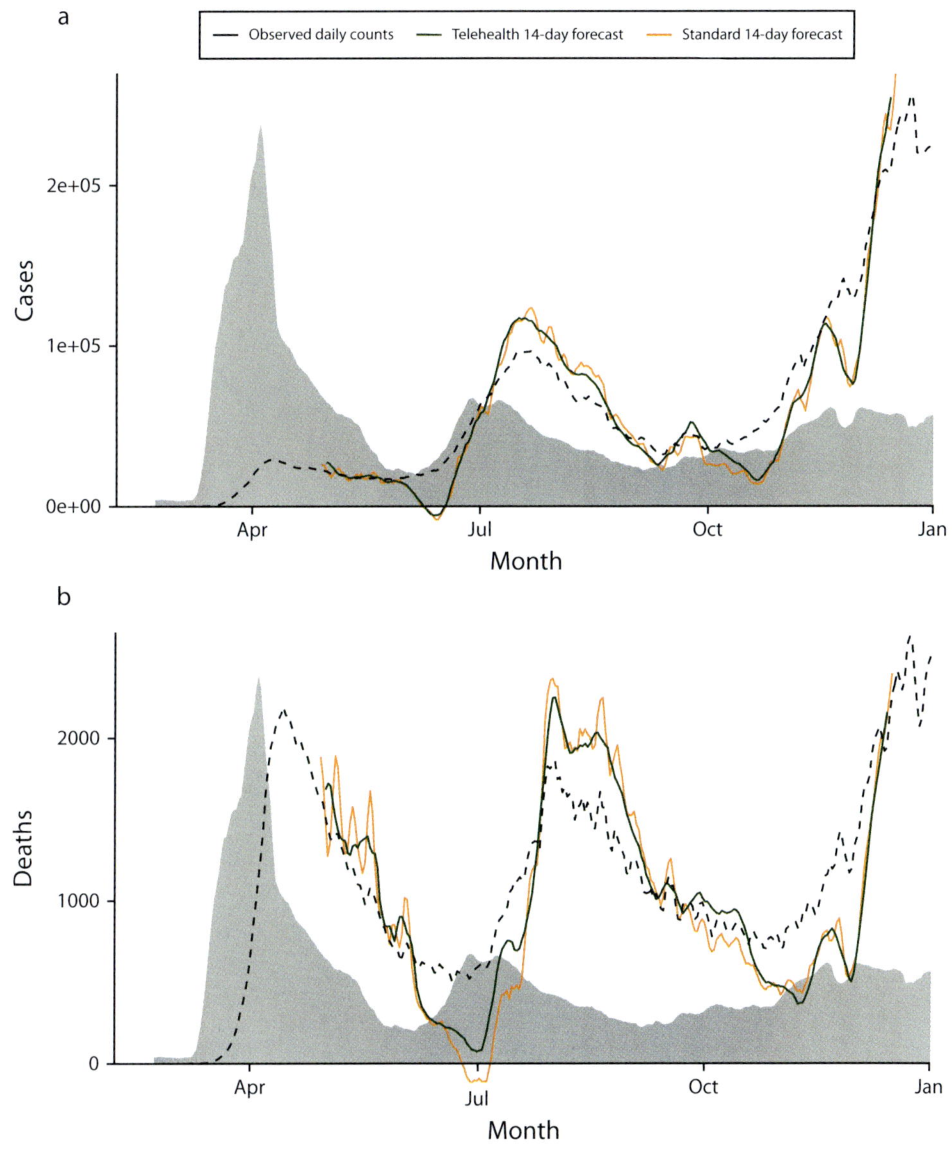

	Mean Absolute Error (SE) of 14-Day Forecasts		Difference (*P*)
	Standard Model	Telehealth Model	
Cases	32.7 (27.22)	30.9 (27.65)	1.8 (<.06)
Deaths	33.3 (27.49)	26.9 (21.13)	6.4 (<.05)

FIGURE 2— Observed Versus Forecasted COVID-19 Cases and Deaths: United States, 2020

guidelines to the provider network, news alerts in-workflow with links to the same guidelines, and rapid changes to the electronic medical record to support physician workflows and repetitive training on new, up-to-date information. Furthermore, this telehealth provider worked with local jurisdictions to support rapid distribution of electronic case reports from within their system. Local jurisdictions establish reporting requirements and rely on case report forms that vary by jurisdiction. Case reporting can optionally leverage the standardized CSTE definitions, which frequently include both laboratory-based criteria and symptom-based case definitions, such as those for influenza-like illness and rheumatic fever.[31]

While there are emerging standards for higher-quality electronic case reports beyond test-confirmed cases,[32] local mandates for case reports vary, and forms and reports are not incorporated into routine health care delivery workflows. If local public health jurisdictions adopt national standards for electronic case reporting,[32–34] both national and local surveillance needs could be efficiently served for high-priority conditions such as COVID-19. Given the market concentration of telehealth urgent-care services, the value of such sources is high compared with implementation costs.

Telehealth-based clinical diagnosis may fill the information gap that rests between traditional health system data and other consumer-based sources that surveillance programs have considered. For example, studies of surveillance based on patients' self-report and search engine symptom entries have generated mixed results, potentially because of endogeneity between public awareness and user-generated activity, but represent another complementary opportunity.[9,11] Information streams based on retail purchases also represent a second level of revealed symptoms, perhaps with fewer confounding issues than self-report or search patterns. Telehealth encounters involve clinician-mediated evaluations not present in self-report or retail data. As acute telehealth encounters disproportionately serve respiratory infections, disseminating CSTE case definitions and collecting data in a unified platform may give dedicated telehealth service providers a distinct and complementary role to existing and contemplated data sources for near-real-time syndromic surveillance information.

Limitations

This study is based on national aggregates of telehealth diagnoses using simplified models that do not include geography, transmission, immunity, or other patient- or population-level characteristics that might further improve model performance to achieve accuracy comparable to previous work.[21] Thus, the absolute values of forecast accuracy measures presented here are conservative estimates. Our results cannot confirm telehealth diagnosis accuracy on a case-wise basis, and true prevalence rates over time are not known, particularly given the asymptomatic spread of COVID-19.[35] In addition, access to this telehealth provider is a common benefit associated with employer-provided health care benefits, and, thus, the population is skewed toward working-age adults, introducing selection bias. While we show here that telehealth-based diagnosis is predictive of future measurements in existing surveillance systems, we cannot rule out additional selection bias similar to existing or alternative surveillance systems that rely on patients seeking or reporting symptom information.

Conclusions

Telehealth-based clinical data may serve as a leading indicator for community spread of emerging infectious disease. Telehealth reports complement other information available to NSSP through in-person services to improve existing surveillance systems. Inclusion of even coarse information from a national dedicated telehealth service provider may add value to existing monitoring and forecasting systems in the future and may warrant infrastructure investments accordingly. AJPH

ABOUT THE AUTHORS

Steven Haenchen, Bridget McCabe, and Jason Tibbels are with Teladoc Health, Purchase, NY. Wendy J. Mack is with Keck School of Medicine, University of Southern California, Los Angeles. Jason N. Doctor is with Schaeffer Center for Health Policy and Economics, University of Southern California. Jeffrey A. Linder and Stephen D. Persell are with Division of General Internal Medicine, Northwestern University Feinberg School of Medicine, Chicago, IL. Daniella Meeker is with Yale School of Medicine, Yale University, New Haven, CT.

CORRESPONDENCE

Correspondence should be sent to Daniella Meeker, PhD, Yale School of Medicine, Yale University, 100 College St, 9th Floor, New Haven, CT 06510 (e-mail: daniella.meeker@yale.edu). Reprints can be ordered at https://ajph.org by clicking the "Reprints" link.

PUBLICATION INFORMATION

Full Citation: Haenchen S, McCabe B, Mack WJ, et al. Use of telehealth information for early detection: insights from the covid-19 pandemic. *Am J Public Health*. 2024;114(2):218–225.

Acceptance Date: October 13, 2023.

DOI: https://doi.org/10.2105/AJPH.2023.307499

CONTRIBUTORS

B. McCabe, D. Meeker, W. J. Mack, and S. Haenchen had full access to all of the data in the study and take responsibility for the integrity of the data and the accuracy of the data analysis. J. A. Linder, S. D. Persell, J. N. Doctor, J. Tibbels, and D. Meeker contributed to concept and design. S. Haenchen, W. J. Mack, and D. Meeker performed the statistical analysis. D. Meeker obtained funding and provided administrative, technical, and material support. B. McCabe and J. A. Linder provided supervision. All authors contributed to acquisition, analysis, or interpretation of data; drafting of the article; and critical revision of the article for important intellectual content.

ACKNOWLEDGMENTS

This project was supported by grant 1R01HS028127-01 from the Agency for Healthcare Research and Quality.

CONFLICTS OF INTEREST

No authors have potential competing nonfinancial or financial conflicts of interest to disclose.

HUMAN PARTICIPANT PROTECTION

The University of Southern California institutional review board approved a waiver of informed consent/assent/parental permission consistent with 45 CFR 46.116(f) on November 21, 2020.

REFERENCES

1. Centers for Disease Control and Prevention. Electronic Surveillance System for the Early Notification of Community-based Epidemics (ESSENCE) operations and maintenance support. Available at: https://sam.gov/opp/7951d04b4cc747bcad0a94dd92f83135/view?index=opp&naics=541&page=3. Accessed November 22, 2021.

2. COVID-19 ForecastHub. About the Hub. Available at: https://covid19forecasthub.org/doc. Accessed November 24, 2021.
3. Burkom H, Loschen W, Wojcik R, et al. Electronic Surveillance System for the Early Notification of Community-Based Epidemics (ESSENCE): overview, components, and public health applications. *JMIR Public Health Surveill.* 2021;7(6):e26303. https://doi.org/10.2196/26303
4. Centers for Disease Control and Prevention. National Syndromic Surveillance Program. Overview. August 19, 2021. Available at: https://www.cdc.gov/nssp/overview.html. Accessed October 24, 2021.
5. Marsden-Haug N, Foster VB, Gould PL, Elbert E, Wang H, Pavlin JA. Code-based syndromic surveillance for influenzalike illness by *International Classification of Diseases, Ninth Revision. Emerg Infect Dis.* 2007;13(2):207–216. https://doi.org/10.3201/eid1302.060557
6. COVID-19 Response Team, Jorden MA, Rudman SL, et al. Evidence for limited early spread of COVID-19 within the United States, January–February 2020. *MMWR Morb Mortal Wkly Rep.* 2020;69(22):680–684. https://doi.org/10.15585/mmwr.mm6922e1
7. Giesecke J. *Modern Infectious Disease Epidemiology.* London, England: CRC Press; 2017.
8. Chan AT, Brownstein JS. Putting the public back in public health—surveying symptoms of Covid-19. *N Engl J Med.* 2020;383(7):e45. https://doi.org/10.1056/NEJMp2016259
9. Lazer D, Kennedy R, King G, Vespignani A. Big data. The parable of Google Flu: traps in big data analysis. *Science.* 2014;343(6176):1203–1205. https://doi.org/10.1126/science.1248506
10. Dugas AF, Jalalpour M, Gel Y, et al. Influenza forecasting with Google Flu Trends. *PLoS One.* 2013;8(2):e56176. https://doi.org/10.1371/journal.pone.0056176
11. Menni C, Valdes AM, Freidin MB, et al. Real-time tracking of self-reported symptoms to predict potential COVID-19. *Nat Med.* 2020;26(7):1037–1040. https://doi.org/10.1038/s41591-020-0916-2
12. Edge VL, Pollari F, Lim G, et al. Syndromic surveillance of gastrointestinal illness using pharmacy over-the-counter sales. *Can J Public Health.* 2004;95(6):446–450. https://doi.org/10.1007/BF03403991
13. Wulandari LPL, Sawitri AAS, Hermansyah A. The potential roles of pharmacy medication sales data to augment the syndromic surveillance system in response to COVID-19 and preparedness for other future infectious disease outbreaks in Indonesia. *Int J Health Plann Manage.* 2021;37(1):30–39. https://doi.org/10.1002/hpm.3356
14. Wharton M, Chorba TL, Vogt RL, Morse DL, Buehler JW. Case definitions for public health surveillance. *MMWR Recomm Rep.* 1990;39(RR-13):1–43.
15. Koonin LM, Hoots B, Tsang CA, et al. Trends in the use of telehealth during the emergence of the COVID-19 pandemic—United States, January–March 2020. *MMWR Morb Mortal Wkly Rep.* 2020;69(43):1595–1599. https://doi.org/10.15585/mmwr.mm6943a3
16. Definitive Healthcare. Top telehealth companies by market share. January 16, 2023. Available at: https://www.definitivehc.com/resources/healthcare-insights/top-telehealth-companies-market-share. Accessed February 3, 2022.
17. Reses HE, Fajans M, Lee SH, et al. Performance of existing and novel surveillance case definitions for COVID-19 in household contacts of PCR-confirmed COVID-19. *BMC Public Health.* 2021;21(1):1747. https://doi.org/10.1186/s12889-021-11683-y
18. Uscher-Pines L, Thompson J, Taylor P, et al. Where virtual care was already a reality: experiences of a nationwide telehealth service provider during the COVID-19 pandemic. *J Med Internet Res.* 2020;22(12):e22727. https://doi.org/10.2196/22727
19. Hoffman DA. Increasing access to care: telehealth during COVID-19. *J Law Biosci.* 2020;7(1):lsaa043. https://doi.org/10.1093/jlb/lsaa043
20. Ray EL, Wattanachit N, Niemi J, et al. Ensemble forecasts of coronavirus disease 2019 (COVID-19) in the U.S. Preprint. Published online August 22, 2020. bioRxiv 20177493. https://doi.org/10.1101/2020.08.19.20177493
21. Cramer EY, Ray EL, Lopez VK, et al. Evaluation of individual and ensemble probabilistic forecasts of COVID-19 mortality in the US. *Proc Natl Acad Sci U S A.* 2022;119(15):e2113561119. https://doi.org/10.1101/2021.02.03.21250974
22. Badr HS, Zaitchik BF, Kerr GH, et al. Unified real-time environmental-epidemiological data for multiscale modeling of the COVID-19 pandemic. *Sci Data.* 2023;10(1):367. https://doi.org/10.1038/s41597-023-02276-y
23. Pinson P. On the predictability of COVID-19. International Institute of Forecasters. September 28, 2021. Available at: https://forecasters.org/blog/2021/09/28/on-the-predictability-of-covid-19. Accessed November 22, 2021.
24. Dong E, Du H, Gardner L. An interactive web-based dashboard to track COVID-19 in real time. *Lancet Infect Dis.* 2020;20(5):533–534. https://doi.org/10.1016/S1473-3099(20)30120-1
25. Health Publications Ltd. *Coronavirus Disease* 2019 (COVID-19): What You Need to Know to Keep Yourself, Your Family, *Pets and Community Safe!* Independently Published; 2020.
26. Cramer EY, Huang Y, Wang Y, et al. The United States COVID-19 Forecast Hub dataset. *Sci Data.* 2022;9(1):462. https://doi.org/10.1038/s41597-022-01517-w
27. Box GEP, Jenkins GM. *Time Series Analysis: Forecasting and Control.* San Francisco, CA: Holden-Day; 1976.
28. Diebold FX, Mariano RS. Comparing predictive accuracy. *J Bus Econ Stat.* 2002;20(1):134–144. https://doi.org/10.1198/073500102753410444
29. US Census Bureau. United States population growth by region. Available at: https://www.census.gov/popclock/print.php?component=growth&image=//www.census.gov/popclock/share/images/growth_1561939200.png. Accessed February 10, 2023.
30. Kiang MV, Irizarry RA, Buckee CO, Balsari S. Every body counts: measuring mortality from the COVID-19 pandemic. *Ann Intern Med.* 2020;173(12):1004–1007. https://doi.org/10.7326/M20-3100
31. Centers for Disease Control and Prevention. Surveillance case definitions for current and historical conditions. Available at: https://ndc.services.cdc.gov. Accessed November 21, 2021.
32. Cooney MA, Iademarco MF, Huang M, MacKenzie WR, Davidson AJ. The public health community platform, electronic case reporting, and the digital bridge. *J Public Health Manag Pract.* 2018;24(2):185–189. https://doi.org/10.1097/PHH.0000000000000775
33. Harris JE. Overcoming reporting delays is critical to timely epidemic monitoring: the case of COVID-19 in New York City. *BMC Public Health.* 2022;22(1):871. https://doi.org/10.1186/s12889-022-13286-7
34. Kissane E, Madrigal A, Anderson J, et al. Assessment of the CDC's new COVID-19 data reporting. Annotated COVID-19 Papers. The Covid Tracking Project. 2020. https://doi.org/10.21428/85acfa8f.54acf4dd
35. Sah P, Fitzpatrick MC, Zimmer CF, et al. Asymptomatic SARS-CoV-2 infection: a systematic review and meta-analysis. *Proc Natl Acad Sci USA.* 2021;118(34):e2109229118. https://doi.org/10.1073/pnas.2109229118

Racial and Ethnic Disaggregation of Tuberculosis Incidence and Risk Factors Among American Indian and Alaska Native Persons—United States, 2001–2020

Yuri P. Springer, PhD, Thomas D. Filardo, MD, Rachel S. Woodruff, MPH, and Julie L. Self, PhD, MPH

See also Cilloni and Dowdy, p. 149.

Objectives. To examine impacts of racial and ethnic disaggregation on the characterization of tuberculosis (TB) epidemiology among American Indian and Alaska Native (AI/AN) persons in the United States.

Methods. Using data reported to the National Tuberculosis Surveillance System during 2001 to 2020, we compared annual age-adjusted TB incidence and the frequency of TB risk factors among 3 AI/AN analytic groups: non-Hispanic AI/AN alone persons, multiracial/Hispanic AI/AN persons, and all AI/AN persons (aggregate of the first 2 groups).

Results. During 2009 to 2020, annual TB incidence (cases per 100 000 persons) among non-Hispanic AI/AN alone persons (range = 3.87–8.56) was on average 1.9 times higher than among all AI/AN persons (range = 1.89–4.70). Compared with non-Hispanic AI/AN alone patients with TB, multiracial/Hispanic AI/AN patients were significantly more likely to be HIV positive (prevalence ratio [PR] = 2.05) and to have been diagnosed while a resident of a correctional facility (PR = 1.71), and significantly less likely to have experienced homelessness (PR = 0.53) or died during TB treatment (PR = 0.47).

Conclusions. Racial and ethnic disaggregation revealed significant differences in TB epidemiology among AI/AN analytic groups. Exclusion of multiracial/Hispanic AI/AN persons from AI/AN analytic groups can substantively affect estimates of racial and ethnic health disparities. (*Am J Public Health*. 2024;114(2): 226–236. https://doi.org/10.2105/AJPH.2023.307498)

Analyses of racial and ethnic health disparities in the United States frequently use a standard classification scheme defined by the US Office of Management and Budget (OMB). The current OMB standard involves aggregating persons with Hispanic ethnicity into a single group irrespective of their race(s) and subsequently classifying persons with non-Hispanic ethnicity into 1 of 5 single-race groups (American Indian or Alaska Native [AI/AN], Asian, Black, Native Hawaiian or other Pacific Islander [NHPI], White) or an aggregate multiracial group.[1] Becker et al. demonstrated that use of the OMB standard may result in inaccurate characterization of health among persons who identify with AI/AN race (hereafter, AI/AN persons) because over 60% of AI/AN persons identify as multiracial or with Hispanic ethnicity and are therefore excluded from the AI/AN OMB group.[2] These exclusions contribute to underestimation of absolute health burdens in AI/AN populations, exacerbating similar effects of AI/AN racial misclassification and incomplete collection of race and ethnicity data that result in chronic undercounting of AI/AN persons by many public health surveillance systems.[2–5] They may also bias characterizations of AI/AN health if

Hispanic or multiracial AI/AN persons differ markedly from non-Hispanic, single-race AI/AN persons in the frequency or outcome of health conditions.

Disaggregation, or the process of breaking down aggregate groups into subgroups, is increasingly utilized to describe racial and ethnic patterns of health more accurately and comprehensively.[6–8] Although racial/ethnic aggregation reduces complexity, it simultaneously masks variation in health characteristics among combined subgroups, thereby obscuring health disparities and complicating the development of tailored health interventions. Through disaggregation, racial and ethnic subgroups can be characterized individually or reaggregated in ways that are more analytically robust, culturally appropriate, and informative to tailored programmatic actions.[2,9–12] The benefits of disaggregation may be especially compelling for AI/AN persons, who constitute a population that is racially and ethnically heterogeneous and relatively small. Large fractions of AI/AN persons are classified into the Hispanic and non-Hispanic multiracial OMB groups, where their contributions to health patterns are essentially made invisible by contributions of demographically larger subgroups. The remaining fraction assigned to the AI/AN OMB group is a minority of all AI/AN persons and thus may not accurately reflect their health; further, the small size of the AI/AN OMB group makes it prone to statistical uncertainty and sensitive to sampling error. In a recent analysis of behavioral and mental health data from the Youth Risk Behavior Survey, Jones and Satter demonstrated how racial/ethnic disaggregation can elucidate variation in health among AI/AN subpopulations.[13]

In the United States, AI/AN persons consistently experience disproportionately high rates of tuberculosis (TB) disease. During 2009 to 2019, mean annual age-adjusted TB incidence among AI/AN persons (6.25 cases per 100 000 persons) was at least 12 times higher than among White persons (0.51 cases per 100 000 persons; both groups comprised US-born, non-Hispanic, single-race persons). In addition, multiple TB risk factors, including diagnosis with diabetes mellitus, diagnosis with end-stage renal disease, and experience of homelessness, occurred at significantly higher frequencies among AI/AN persons with TB.[14] These health disparities highlight the particular importance of interventions to control TB among AI/AN persons.

We applied racial and ethnic disaggregation to describe more comprehensively and accurately the epidemiology of TB disease among AI/AN persons in the United States during 2001 to 2020. We estimated annual disease incidence and the frequency of various clinical and sociobehavioral characteristics separately for (1) non-Hispanic, single-race AI/AN persons and (2) Hispanic and multiracial AI/AN persons with TB to examine how the TB-related health profiles of these 2 AI/AN subpopulations differed. Additionally, we estimated incidence and frequency of characteristics among all persons with TB who identified with AI/AN race (i.e., irrespective of their ethnicity or identification with other race[s]) to evaluate how use of a more racially and ethnically inclusive AI/AN group definition would affect estimates of TB-related disparities compared with those typically reported for the AI/AN OMB group. Our findings demonstrate how the selection of race and ethnicity groups for stratified analyses of health data can influence descriptions of epidemiological patterns and health disparities and can facilitate characterization of racial and ethnic subpopulations for the development of tailored health interventions.

METHODS

We analyzed data on all incident cases of TB disease reported to the Centers for Disease Control and Prevention's National Tuberculosis Surveillance System (NTSS) that met the case definition[15] during January 1, 2001 to December 31, 2020 and were counted within any of the 50 states or the District of Columbia. Using self-reported race and ethnicity data, we assigned cases to 1 or 2 of 4 race/ethnicity groups: cases in persons with TB (hereafter "patients" for brevity) who identified with (1) AI/AN race alone and with non-Hispanic ethnicity (hereafter "non-Hispanic AI/AN alone"), (2) AI/AN race in combination with 1 or more other races and with non-Hispanic ethnicity or with AI/AN race (alone or in combination with 1 or more other races) and with Hispanic ethnicity (hereafter "multiple/Hispanic AI/AN"), (3) AI/AN race (i.e., either alone or in combination with 1 or more other races and with either Hispanic or non-Hispanic ethnicity; hereafter "all AI/AN"), and (4) White race alone and with non-Hispanic ethnicity (hereafter "non-Hispanic White alone"; Table 1). Note that the all AI/AN group includes all cases assigned to the non-Hispanic AI/AN alone and multiple/Hispanic AI/AN groups. The non-Hispanic AI/AN alone and non-Hispanic White alone groups are identical to those used in the OMB standard[1]; they are commonly used to represent AI/AN and White persons in the United States.

AJPH February 2024, Vol. 114, No. 2

TABLE 1— Counts and Percentages of Reported Tuberculosis (TB) Cases by Patient Race and Ethnicity: United States, 2001–2020

	Ethnicity, No. (%)		
Race	**Non-Hispanic**	**Hispanic**	**Unknown**
AI/AN			
Single race	2 709 (82.5)[a]	373 (11.4)[b]	20 (0.6)
Multiracial	143 (4.4)[b]	39 (1.2)[b]	1 (0.0)
Asian			
Single race	64 306 (98.4)[a]	367 (0.6)	61 (0.1)
Multiracial	562 (0.9)	29 (0.0)	0 (0.0)
Black			
Single race	57 015 (96.8)[a]	1 488 (2.5)	70 (0.1)
Multiracial	271 (0.5)	63 (0.1)	1 (0.0)
NHPI			
Single race	1 593 (89.2)[a]	48 (2.7)	1 (0.1)
Multiracial	131 (7.3)	11 (0.6)	2 (0.1)
White			
Single race	36 859 (37.0)[a]	61 945 (62.2)	47 (0.0)
Multiracial	567 (0.6)	186 (0.2)	0 (0.0)
Unknown/missing race[c]			
Single race	325 (23.3)	748 (53.7)	77 (5.5)
Multiracial	158 (11.4)	84 (6.0)	0 (0.0)
Overall			
Single race	162 482 (70.6)	64 221 (27.9)	199 (0.1)
Multiracial	1 832 (0.8)	412 (0.2)	4 (0.0)
Unknown race	325 (0.1)	748 (0.3)	77 (0.0)

Note. AI/AN = American Indian or Alaska Native; NHPI = Native Hawaiian or Other Pacific Islander. Counts represent the number of race/ethnicity endorsements by patients with TB, not necessarily the number of TB cases. Total count of table records is 230 300 but total number of cases during this time period was 229 164; totals are discrepant because multiracial patients with TB make multiple race/ethnicity endorsements and are thus counted more than once. Percentages may total greater than 100%. Percentages were calculated relative to the total number of race/ethnicity endorsements associated with each of the 6 race categories.

[a]Denotes race/ethnicity combinations commonly used to represent AI/AN, Asian, Black, NHPI, and White persons according to reporting standards set forth by the US Office of Management and Budget.[1]

[b]Denotes race/ethnicity combinations that constitute the multiple/Hispanic AI/AN race/ethnicity group in this investigation.

[c]When unknown race was reported in combination with at least 1 other race, that patient with TB was classified as multiracial even though 1 of their races was unspecified.

We stratified all analyses by race/ethnicity group. We calculated annual age-adjusted TB incidence (per 100 000 persons) during 2009 to 2020 using population estimates from the US Census Bureau's American Community Survey 5-year public use microdata sample (PUMS) data set[16]; 2009 was the earliest year for which the requisite data were available in the data set. We performed age adjustment using direct standardization to the 2010 US population, as this year was near the temporal midpoint of our investigation.[17] We calculated associated 95% confidence intervals using the log Student's *t* method,[18] with variance of incidence based on PUMS person-weights. We visualized temporal trends in incidence using 5-year centered moving averages. We compared annual incidence among groups using incidence rate ratios; we calculated associated 95% confidence intervals using the normal approximation (Wald) method. We used the non-Hispanic White alone and multiple/Hispanic groups as references, the former because it consistently has the lowest annual TB incidence among race/ethnicity groups[15] and the latter for direct comparison with the non-Hispanic AI/AN alone group. We similarly compared the characteristics of patients with TB during 2001 to 2020 using prevalence ratios and 95% confidence intervals or using χ^2 tests. We calculated 95% confidence intervals using the normal approximation (Wald) method if the numerator for the nonreference group was greater than 10; otherwise, we used a bootstrap method with 10 000 replicates. We defined statistical significance as $P < .05$. We identified TB cases attributed to recent transmission during 2011 to 2020 using the plausible source-case method[19] and tuberculosis genotyping data obtained by spoligotyping and 24 locus mycobacterial interspersed repetitive units variable number of tandem repeats (MIRU-VNTR) molecular typing methods. Because sputum culture isolates needed for genotyping *Mycobacterium tuberculosis* cannot be consistently obtained from younger patients, we only considered cases in patients aged 15 years or older when evaluating data on recent transmission.

RESULTS

During 2009 to 2020, the number of persons in the United States who identified with AI/AN race (i.e., the all AI/AN group) ranged from 4 581 897 (2009) to 5 757 592 (2020)[16] (Table A, available as a supplement to the online version of this article at http://www.ajph.org). Of these persons, the annual percentage that identified with AI/AN race alone and with non-Hispanic ethnicity (i.e., the non-Hispanic AI/AN alone group) decreased consistently over time, from 44.4% (2009) to 35.9% (2020). By comparison, the annual percentage that identified with AI/AN race in combination with 1 or more other races and with non-Hispanic ethnicity or with AI/AN race (either alone or in combination with 1 or more other races) and with Hispanic ethnicity (i.e., the multiple/Hispanic AI/AN group) increased consistently over time, from 55.6% (2009) to 64.1% (2020)[16] (Table A). Among persons in this multiple/Hispanic AI/AN group, an annual mean of 33.6% identified as Hispanic AI/AN (range = 29.2%–38.2%) and 66.4% identified as non-Hispanic multiracial AI/AN persons (range = 61.8%–70.8%).

Of the 229 164 incident TB cases reported to the NTSS during 2001 to 2020, 3264 (1.4%) were in patients who identified with AI/AN race and either Hispanic or non-Hispanic ethnicity. Among these, 2709 (82.5%) identified as non-Hispanic AI/AN alone, 373 (11.4%) identified as Hispanic AI/AN alone, 143 (4.4%) identified as non-Hispanic AI/AN in combination with 1 or more other races, and 39 (1.2%) identified as Hispanic AI/AN in combination with 1 or more other races (Table 1). Ethnicity data were missing for 21 (0.6%) patients who identified with AI/AN race (20 AI/AN alone, 1 AI/AN in combination with 1 or more other races).

Tuberculosis Incidence

Age-adjusted annual TB incidence (per 100 000 persons) was significantly higher for the non-Hispanic AI/AN alone group (mean = 6.05; range = 3.87–8.56) than for the multiple/Hispanic AI/AN group (mean = 1.07; range = 0.60–1.86) in all years; values for the all AI/AN group were intermediate in all years (mean = 3.15; range = 1.89–4.70; by comparison, for the non-Hispanic White alone group, mean = 0.60; range = 0.35–0.85; Figure A, Table B, available as a supplement to the online version of this article at http://www.ajph.org). The plot of 5-year centered moving averages of age-adjusted annual incidence showed that values for both groups decreased over time (Figure 1). Relative to the non-Hispanic White alone group, age-adjusted annual incidence rate ratios ranged from 7.03 to 13.25 for the non-Hispanic AI/AN alone group and from 1.27 to 2.28 for the multiple/Hispanic AI/AN group; the plot of associated 5-year moving averages showed that values for both groups were relatively consistent over the investigation period (Figure 1, Figure A, Table B). When we compared incidence for the non-Hispanic AI/AN alone and multiple/Hispanic AI/AN groups, age-adjusted annual incidence rate ratios for the latter ranged from 0.10 to 0.31 (Figure 1, Figure A, Table B). Results based on crude annual TB incidence and associated incidence rate ratios were qualitatively similar (Figure B, Figure C, Table C, available as a supplement to the online version of this article at http://www.ajph.org).

Patient Characteristics

Multiple/Hispanic AI/AN patients compared with non-Hispanic AI/AN alone patients. Relative to non-Hispanic AI/AN alone patients with TB, a significantly higher percentage of multiple/Hispanic AI/AN patients were younger than 45 years (61.6% vs 40.8%; $\chi^2 = 81.3$) and resided in the South Atlantic (26.7% vs 7.0%; $\chi^2 = 192.9$) and Middle Atlantic (6.7% vs 0.4%; $\chi^2 = 128.7$) Census Divisions[20]; a significantly lower percentage resided in the Mountain Census Division (3.8% vs 26.4%; $\chi^2 = 134.5$) and were diagnosed based on positive culture (74.6% vs 82.6%; $\chi^2 = 11.8$; all comparisons, $P < .001$; Table D, available as a supplement to the online version of this article at http://www.ajph.org).

Among the subset of patients with TB aged 15 years or older, multiple/Hispanic AI/AN patients were significantly more likely than non-Hispanic AI/AN alone patients to have been HIV positive at diagnosis (prevalence ratio [PR] = 2.05) and to have been a resident of a correctional facility at the time of their current TB episode (PR = 1.71; Figure 2,Table D, Table E, available as a supplement to the online version of this article at http://www.ajph.org). Multiple/Hispanic AI/AN patients were significantly less likely to have reported using alcohol to excess (PR = 0.41), experiencing homelessness (PR = 0.53), being primarily unemployed (PR = 0.58), or using noninjection drugs (PR = 0.75) during the 12 months prior to TB diagnosis; they were also less likely to have their current episode of TB disease attributed to recent transmission (PR = 0.48). Among patients with TB of all ages, multiple/Hispanic AI/AN patients were significantly more likely than non-Hispanic AI/AN alone patients to have had cavitary disease on chest radiograph or chest computed tomography scan (PR = 1.22) and were significantly less likely to have died during TB treatment (PR = 0.47) or experienced TB disease previously (PR = 0.52; Figure 2, Table D, Table E).

All AI/AN patients compared with non-Hispanic White alone patients. When we compared the frequencies of patient characteristics between the all AI/AN and non-Hispanic White alone groups, observed differences were driven largely by non-Hispanic AI/AN alone patients, with inclusion of multiple/Hispanic AI/AN patients exerting relatively modest effects. Of the 19 characteristics evaluated, 15 occurred at significantly different frequencies among all AI/AN and non-Hispanic White alone patients. Of these, 8 occurred significantly more frequently among non-Hispanic AI/AN alone and all AI/AN patients but not among multiple/Hispanic AI/AN patients. These included having the current episode of TB disease attributed to recent transmission (PR = 2.78 for non-Hispanic AI/AN alone patients, PR = 2.52 for all AI/AN patients), being diagnosed with end-stage renal disease or chronic renal failure (PR = 2.10 and PR = 1.96), and reporting using alcohol to excess (PR = 2.09 and PR = 1.89) and experiencing homelessness (PR = 2.02 and PR = 1.86) during the 12 months prior to TB diagnosis (all characteristics among patients aged ≥ 15 years; Figure 3, Table D, Table E). By comparison, only 3 of the 15 characteristics occurred significantly more or less frequently among multiple/Hispanic AI/AN and all AI/AN patients (compared with non-Hispanic White alone patients) but not among non-Hispanic AI/AN alone patients: being a resident of a correctional facility at the time of the

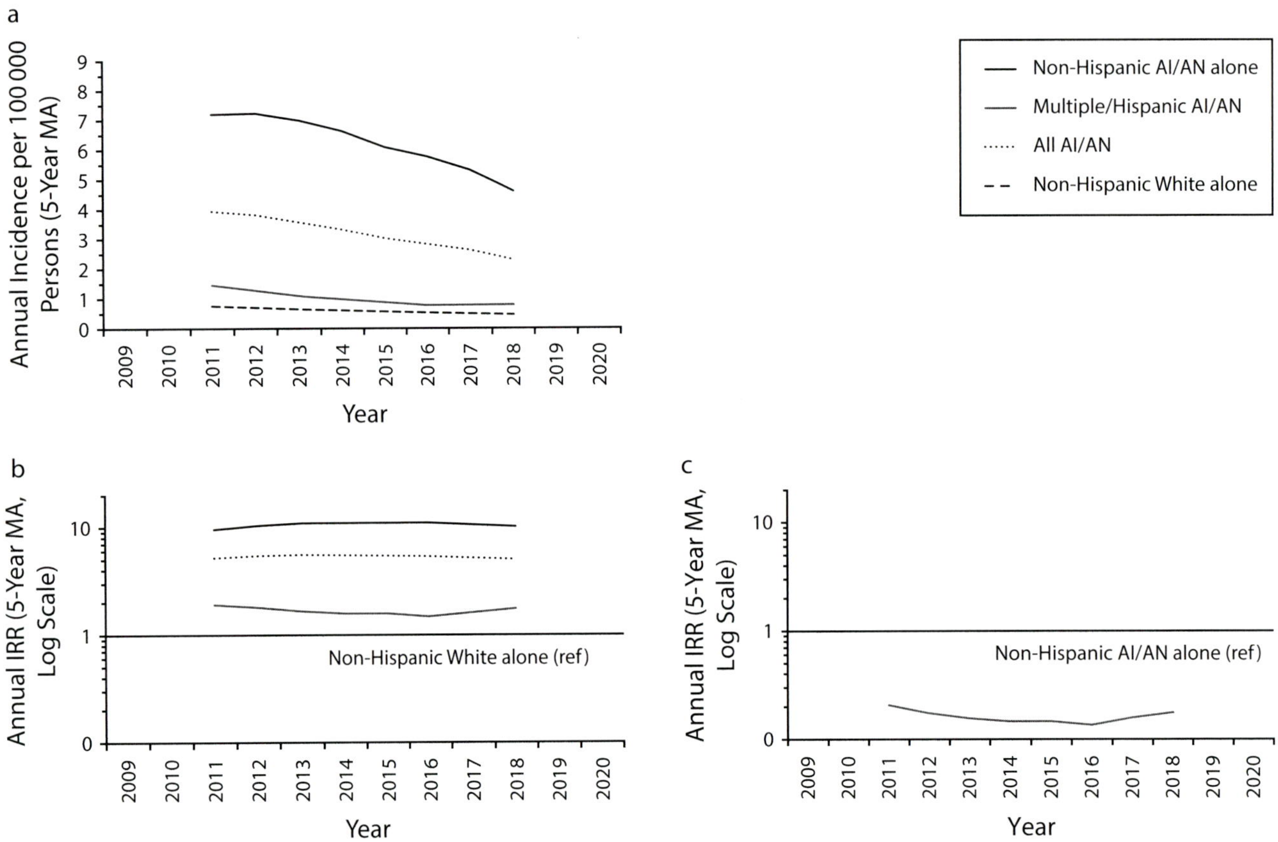

FIGURE 1— Age-Adjusted Annual Tuberculosis (a) 5-Year Centered Moving Averages, and Associated Incidence Rate Ratios for (b) the Non-Hispanic AI/AN Alone, Multiple/Hispanic AI/AN, and All AI/AN vs Non-Hispanic White Alone Race/Ethnicity Groups and (c) Multiple/Hispanic AI/AN vs Non-Hispanic AI/AN Alone Race/Ethnicity Groups: United States, 2009–2020

Note. AI/AN = American Indian/Alaska Native; IRR = incidence rate ratio; MA = moving average. Note that in parts b and c, IRR values are plotted on a log scale. Case counts were based on self-reported race/ethnicity. The non-Hispanic AI/AN alone and non-Hispanic White alone race/ethnicity groups include single-race, non-Hispanic AI/AN or White persons, respectively. The multiple/Hispanic AI/AN race/ethnicity group includes multiracial non-Hispanic AI/AN persons and single-race or multiracial Hispanic AI/AN persons. The all AI/AN group included all AI/AN persons (single race and multiracial, Hispanic and non-Hispanic).
Source. Age-adjusted incidence calculated using population estimates from the US Census Bureau's American Community Survey (ACS) 5-year public use microdata sample (PUMS) data set[16] and direct standardization to the 2010 US population.[17]

current TB episode (among patients aged ≥ 15 years, PR = 1.99 for multiple/Hispanic AI/AN patients and PR = 1.30 for all AI/AN patients), having cavitary disease (PR = 1.25 and PR = 1.06), and having any pulmonary disease (PR = 0.93 and PR = 0.97; Figure 3, Table D, Table E). The remaining 4 of 15 characteristics occurred significantly more or less frequently among both non-Hispanic AI/AN alone and multiple/Hispanic AI/AN patients, and thus by extension among all AI/AN patients (compared with non-Hispanic White alone patients): reporting use of noninjection drugs during the 12 months prior to TB diagnosis, being diagnosed with diabetes mellitus, being immunosuppressed because of a condition other than HIV/AIDS or a medication, and receiving treatment of the current TB episode partially or completely as directly observed therapy (all but the last characteristic among patients aged ≥ 15 years).

DISCUSSION

Our analyses applying racial and ethnic disaggregation to data on TB in AI/AN persons generated 2 principal findings. First, inclusion of data on multiple/Hispanic AI/AN persons significantly decreased estimated TB incidence in the all AI/AN group relative to the non-Hispanic AI/AN alone group. Second, although analyses of patient characteristics identified unique attributes of multiple/Hispanic AI/AN patients with TB, these were largely masked in the all AI/AN group by patterns associated with the non-Hispanic AI/AN alone group. Both results were strongly influenced by the differing contributions of non-Hispanic AI/AN alone and multiple/Hispanic AI/AN persons to the number of TB cases among AI/AN persons and the size of the general AI/AN population. These findings

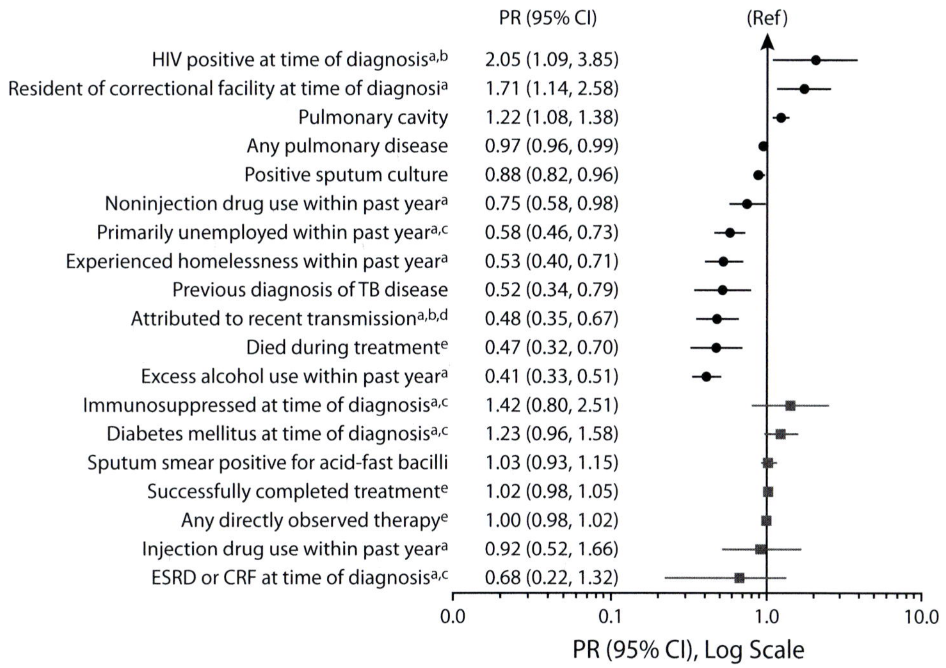

FIGURE 2— Prevalence of Patient Characteristics for Tuberculosis (TB) Cases Assigned to the Multiple/Hispanic AI/AN Race/Ethnicity Group Compared With Cases Assigned to the Non-Hispanic AI/AN Alone Race/Ethnicity Group: United States, 2001–2020

Note. AI/AN = American Indian/Alaska Native; CI = confidence interval; CRF = chronic renal failure; ESRD = end-stage renal disease; PR = prevalence ratio. Case counts are based on self-reported race/ethnicity. The non-Hispanic AI/AN alone group includes single-race, non-Hispanic AI/AN persons. The multiple/Hispanic AI/AN group includes multiracial non-Hispanic AI/AN persons and single-race or multiracial Hispanic AI/AN persons. PRs and 95% CIs were calculated by using the normal approximation (Wald) method when the numerator for the nonreference group PR was > 10 and otherwise using a bootstrap method with 10 000 replicates. Black circles denote statistically significant PRs ($P < .05$); gray squares denote non-significant PRs. For details about the data categories compared for each characteristic, see Tables D and E (available as a supplement to the online version of this article at http://www.ajph.org).

[a]Among patients with TB aged ≥ 15 years.

[b]During 2011–2020 only.

[c]During 2010–2020 only.

[d]Using the plausible source-case method[19] and molecular surveillance data generated using spoligotyping and 24 locus mycobacterial interspersed repetitive units variable number of tandem repeats (MIRU-VNTR) molecular typing methods to identify TB cases attributable to recent transmission.

[e]During 2001–2018 only.

demonstrate how decisions involving inclusion criteria for analytic race/ethnicity groups can substantively affect estimates of the nature and magnitude of health disparities.

Among our 3 AI/AN race/ethnicity groups, TB incidence rates were consistently highest for the non-Hispanic AI/AN alone group; this is the group typically used to represent AI/AN persons in analyses stratified by race and ethnicity and to report associated health disparities. The mean annual age-adjusted incidence for this group was 10.2 times that for the non-Hispanic White alone group (mean annual absolute difference = 5.4 cases per 100 000 persons). By comparison, rates were consistently lowest for the multiple/Hispanic AI/AN group; the mean annual age-adjusted incidence was 82% lower than for the non-Hispanic AI/AN alone group (mean annual absolute difference = 5.0 cases per 100 000). This difference resulted from the fact that the non-Hispanic AI/AN alone group accounted on average for 79% of the annual number of TB cases in the all AI/AN group but only 40% of that group's population. Thus, combining the non-Hispanic AI/AN alone and multiple/Hispanic AI/AN groups to create the all AI/AN group resulted in intermediate rates; mean annual age-adjusted incidence for the all AI/AN group was only 5.2 times that for the non-Hispanic White alone group (mean annual absolute difference of 2.6 cases per 100 000 persons). The magnitude of the

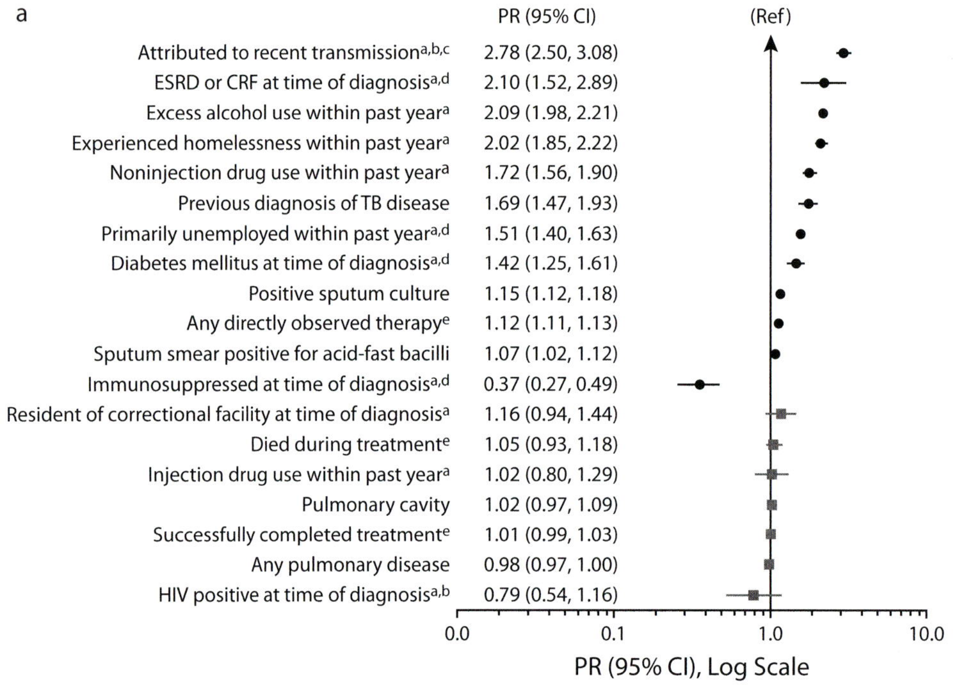

FIGURE 3— Prevalence of Patient Characteristics for Tuberculosis (TB) Cases Assigned to (a) the Non-Hispanic AI/AN Alone Race/Ethnicity Group, (b) the Multiple/Hispanic AI/AN Race/Ethnicity Group, and (c) the All AI/AN Race/Ethnicity Group Compared With Cases Assigned to the Non-Hispanic White Alone Race/Ethnicity Group: United States, 2001–2020

Note. AI/AN = American Indian/Alaska Native; CI = confidence interval; CRF = chronic renal failure; ESRD = end-stage renal disease; PR = prevalence ratio; Ref = non-Hispanic White alone. PR values are plotted on a log scale. Case counts were based on self-reported race/ethnicity. Non-Hispanic AI/AN alone and Non-Hispanic White alone groups include single-race, non-Hispanic AI/AN or White persons, respectively. Multiple/Hispanic AI/AN group includes multiracial non-Hispanic AI/AN persons and single-race or multiracial Hispanic AI/AN persons. All AI/AN group includes all AI/AN persons (single race and multiracial, Hispanic and non-Hispanic). PRs and 95% CIs were calculated by using the normal approximation (Wald) method when the numerator for the nonreference group PR was > 10 and otherwise using a bootstrap method with 10 000 replicates. Black circles denote statistically significant PRs ($P < .05$); gray squares denote non-significant PRs. For details about the data categories compared for each characteristic, see Tables D and E (available as a supplement to the online version of this article at http://www.ajph.org).

[a]Among patients with TB aged ≥ 15 years.
[b]During 2011–2020 only.
[c]Using the plausible source-case method[19] and molecular surveillance data generated using spoligotyping and 24 locus mycobacterial interspersed repetitive units variable number of tandem repeats (MIRU-VNTR) molecular typing methods to identify TB cases attributable to recent transmission.
[d]ESRD: end-stage renal disease; CRF: chronic renal failure.
[e]During 2010–2020 only.
[f]During 2001–2018 only.

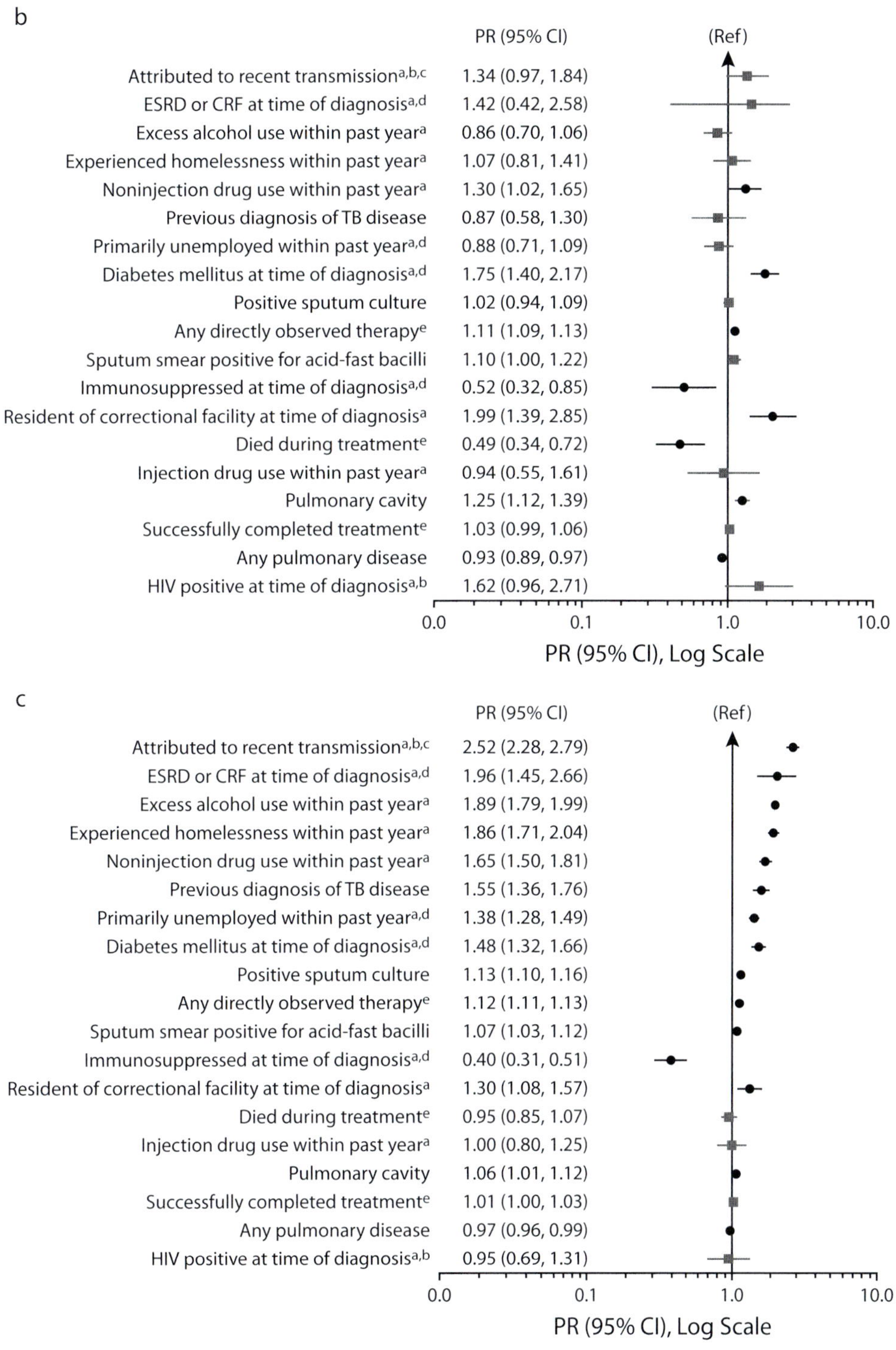

FIGURE 3— Continued

disparity in TB incidence typically associated with AI/AN persons based on a comparison of the AI/AN OMB group (i.e., non-Hispanic AI/AN alone group) to the non-Hispanic White alone group was reduced by approximately 50% by broadening group inclusion criteria to include Hispanic and multiracial AI/AN persons.

Analyses of patient characteristics similarly evidenced the disproportionate representation of non-Hispanic AI/AN alone persons among all AI/AN

TB cases. The patient characteristics profile for the all AI/AN group was nearly identical to that of the non-Hispanic AI/AN alone group. Relative to TB in patients in the non-Hispanic White alone group, TB among patients in the all AI/AN group was associated with significantly elevated frequencies of various epidemiological (e.g., having the current episode of TB disease attributed to recent transmission, having a previous TB diagnosis), clinical (e.g., diagnosis with end-stage renal disease or chronic renal failure or diabetes), and sociobehavioral risk factors (e.g., use of alcohol to excess, use of noninjection drugs, experience of homelessness, or being primarily unemployed within the previous year). Separate evaluation of patients in the multiple/Hispanic AI/AN group identified several distinctive characteristics relative to patients in the non-Hispanic AI/AN alone group, including significantly lower frequencies of all of the aforementioned epidemiological and sociobehavioral risk factors. Compared with non-Hispanic AI/AN alone patients with TB, multiple/Hispanic AI/AN patients were significantly more likely to be HIV positive, be a resident of a correctional facility, have cavitary disease, and reside in the South and Middle Atlantic Census Regions (where they accounted for nearly half of all AI/AN TB cases). Identification of these distinct patient characteristic profiles illustrates how analyses employing racial/ethnic disaggregation can inform the development of public health interventions tailored to epidemiologically distinct patient subpopulations.

In analyses of health data stratified by race and ethnicity, non-Hispanic single-race OMB standard groups are commonly used to represent all persons of a particular race. Setting aside considerations of the cultural appropriateness and acceptability of this approach and evaluating it strictly through a quantitative lens, the former will be a reasonable proxy for the latter when the number and population fraction of excluded persons (i.e., those who identify as multiracial or with Hispanic ethnicity) are small. For example, during 2001 to 2020, the non-Hispanic single race OMB standard Asian and Black groups excluded 1.5% and 3.1% of TB cases involving patients who identified with Asian race and with Black race, respectively (Table 1). In contrast, the non-Hispanic single race OMB standard AI/AN group excluded 17% of TB cases involving patients who identified with AI/AN race. These findings parallel demographic proportions observed in the general population. During 2016 to 2020, non-Hispanic, single-race persons accounted for an annual average of 83% and 88% of persons who identified with Asian and Black race, respectively, but only 38% of persons who identified with AI/AN race (Table F, available as a supplement to the online version of this article at http://www.ajph.org). Among these AI/AN persons, 52% and 22% identified as multiracial and with Hispanic ethnicity, respectively. Trend analyses using data from the US Census Bureau and Pew Research Center surveys suggest that the sizes of these multiracial and Hispanic population fractions are likely to increase across all race groups in coming years.[21,22] Thus, application of racial/ethnic disaggregation and use of analytic groups that are more inclusive than those currently defined by the OMB will become increasingly necessary to accurately characterize racial and ethnic patterns of health, particularly for AI/AN persons.

This investigation had at least 2 general limitations. The quality of underlying data could have been reduced by racial/ethnic misclassification, a problem of particular concern for AI/AN persons.[2,4] NTSS reporting guidelines specify that race and ethnicity data should be collected by patient self-report, which should minimize misclassification rates, yet reporting biases may persist, and in some instances these data may be gathered from other sources that may not capture self-reported data (e.g., electronic health records). Additionally, our analyses of patient characteristics did not control for variation in the frequencies of risk factors in underlying populations.

Our findings serve as a reminder that measurements of health disparities are not absolute, but instead reflect the particular groups chosen for comparison. Despite pervasive use, OMB standard groups are merely generalized administrative constructs intended to standardize reporting of data stratified by race and ethnicity. There is no singularly correct or even universally accepted definition of racial and ethnic identification because notions of what define a person of a particular race or ethnicity are highly subjective and vary among populations, communities, and even for individuals over time.[23] Racial and ethnic identification may be especially nuanced for persons who identify with AI/AN race as they constitute a population characterized by a uniquely complex intersectionality of high and rising rates of multiracial association, ethnic diversity, tribal affiliation, and urban versus rural partitioning.[24] Consistent with the subjectivity of racial and ethnic identification, work to characterize racial and ethnic health disparities should include thoughtful, inclusive, culturally sensitive selection of analytic groups, explicit articulation of associated selection criteria, clear attribution of findings to selected groups and associated (sub)populations, and consideration and evaluation of how use of alternative groups might have influenced findings, conclusions, and recommendations. By applying disaggregation and measuring differences in the health of groups defined in multiple ways, investigations of racial and ethnic health disparities can provide quantitative insight into uncertainty associated with differences among groups akin to a sensitivity analysis. This analytic approach can contribute to more accurate and precise characterization of the nature and magnitude of health disparities and thereby inform more effectively tailored interventions to promote health equity. AJPH

ABOUT THE AUTHORS

Yuri P. Springer, Thomas D. Filardo, Rachel S. Woodruff, and Julie L. Self are with the Centers for Disease Control and Prevention, National Center for HIV, Viral Hepatitis, STD, and TB Prevention, Division of Tuberculosis Elimination, Atlanta, GA. Thomas D. Filardo is also with the Epidemic Intelligence Service, Centers for Disease Control and Prevention, National Center for State, Tribal, Local, and Territorial Public Health Infrastructure and Workforce, Division of Workforce Development, Atlanta, GA.

CORRESPONDENCE

Correspondence should be sent to Yuri P. Springer, 1600 Clifton Rd NE, Atlanta, GA 30329 (e-mail: vkh3@cdc.gov). Reprints can be ordered at http://www.ajph.org by clicking the "Reprints" link.

PUBLICATION INFORMATION

Full Citation: Springer YP, Filardo TD, Woodruff RS, Self JL. Racial and ethnic disaggregation of tuberculosis incidence and risk factors among american indian and alaska native persons—united states, 2001–2020. *Am J Public Health*. 2024; 114(2):226–236.

Acceptance Date: October 12, 2023.

DOI: https://doi.org/10.2105/AJPH.2023.307498

ORCID iDs:

Julie L. Self https://orcid.org/0000-0001-9584-7041

CONTRIBUTORS

Y. P. Springer conceptualized the investigation. Y. P. Springer and T. D. Filardo led the analyses and writing and contributed equally to the work. All authors contributed to analyses and writing and approved the final manuscript.

ACKNOWLEDGMENTS

This work was funded by the Centers for Disease Control and Prevention. Excluding staff hours, no funds were allocated specifically for this investigation.

We thank S. E. Jones for insights and encouragement shared during the conceptualization of this investigation, K. Irimata for assistance with statistical analyses, and all public health staff who contribute data to the National Tuberculosis Surveillance System.

Note. The findings and conclusions in this report are those of the authors and do not necessarily represent the official position of the Centers for Disease Control and Prevention (CDC).

CONFLICTS OF INTEREST

The authors declare that they have no relevant financial or nonfinancial conflicts of interest to disclose.

HUMAN PARTICIPANT PROTECTION

This work was determined not to constitute human subjects research by the Centers for Disease Control and Prevention and did not require approval by an institutional review board because data were collected and analyzed as part of routine public health surveillance.

REFERENCES

1. Office of Management and Budget. Revisions to the standards for the classification of federal data on race and ethnicity. *Fed Regist*. 1997; 62(210):58782–58790.
2. Becker T, Babey SH, Dorsey R, Ponce NA. Data disaggregation with American Indian/Alaska Native population data. *Popul Res Policy Rev*. 2021;40(1):103–125. https://doi.org/10.1007/s11113-020-09635-2
3. Hatcher SM, Agnew-Brune C, Anderson M, et al. COVID-19 among American Indian and Alaska Native persons—23 states, January 31–July 3, 2020. *MMWR Morb Mortal Wkly Rep*. 2020;69(34): 1166–1169. https://doi.org/10.15585/mmwr.mm6934e1
4. Jim MA, Arias E, Seneca DS, et al. Racial misclassification of American Indians and Alaska Natives by Indian Health Service contract health service delivery area. *Am J Public Health*. 2014;104(suppl 3):S295–S302. https://doi.org/10.2105/AJPH.2014.301933
5. Mays VM, Echo-Hawk A, Cochran SD, Akee R. Data equity in American Indian/Alaska Native populations: respecting sovereign nations' right to meaningful and usable COVID-19 data. *Am J Public Health*. 2022;112(10):1416–1420. https://doi.org/10.2105/AJPH.2022.307043
6. Gigli KH. Data disaggregation: a research tool to identify health inequities. *J Pediatr Health Care*. 2021;35(3):332–336. https://doi.org/10.1016/j.pedhc.2020.12.002
7. Kauh TJ. Read JnG, Scheitler A. The critical role of racial/ethnic data disaggregation for health equity. *Popul Res Policy Rev*. 2021;40(1):1–7. https://doi.org/10.1007/s11113-020-09631-6
8. Rubin V, Ngo D, Ross A, Butler D, Balaram N. Counting a diverse nation: disaggregating data on race and ethnicity to advance a culture of health. 2018. Available at: https://www.policylink.org/resources-tools/counting-a-diverse-nation. Accessed May 3, 2023.
9. Alcántara C, Suglia SF, Ibarra IP, et al. Disaggregation of Latina/o child and adult health data: a systematic review of public health surveillance surveys in the United States. *Popul Res Policy Rev*. 2021;40(1):61–79. https://doi.org/10.1007/s11113-020-09633-4
10. Larimore S, Ifatunji M, Lee H, Rafferty J, Jackson J, Hicken MT. Geographic variation in reproductive health among the black population in the US: an analysis of nativity, region of origin, and division of residence. *Popul Res Policy Rev*. 2021; 40(1):33–59. https://doi.org/10.1007/s11113-020-09629-0
11. Read JG, Lynch SM, West JS. Disaggregating heterogeneity among non-Hispanic whites: evidence and implications for US racial/ethnic health disparities. *Popul Res Policy Rev*. 2021; 40(1):9–31. https://doi.org/10.1007/s11113-020-09632-5
12. Shimkhada R, Scheitler A, Ponce NA. Capturing racial/ethnic diversity in population-based surveys: data disaggregation of health data for Asian American, Native Hawaiian, and Pacific Islanders (AANHPIs). *Popul Res Policy Rev*. 2021;40(1): 81–102. https://doi.org/10.1007/s11113-020-09634-3
13. Jones SE, Satter DE. Implications for coding race and ethnicity for American Indian and Alaska Native high school students in a national survey. *J Health Care Poor Underserved*. 2022;33(3): 1245–1257. https://doi.org/10.1353/hpu.2022.0110
14. Springer YP, Kammerer JS, Silk BJ, Langer AJ. Tuberculosis in indigenous persons—United States, 2009–2019. *J Racial Ethn Health Disparities*. 2022; 5(9):1750–1764.
15. Centers for Disease Control and Prevention. Reported tuberculosis in the United States, 2021. Available at: https://www.cdc.gov/tb/statistics/reports/2021/default.htm. Accessed May 3, 2023.
16. US Census Bureau. American Community Survey (ACS) 5-year public use microdata samples. Available at: https://data.census.gov/mdat/#. Accessed May 3, 2023.
17. Li C, Ford ES, Zhao G, Wen XJ, Gotway CA. Age adjustment of diabetes prevalence: use of 2010 US Census data. *J Diabetes*. 2014;6(5): 451–461. https://doi.org/10.1111/1753-0407.12122
18. Parker JD, Talih M, Irimata KE, et al. National Center for Health Statistics data presentation standards for rates and counts. *Vital Health Stat*. 2023;2(200):1–26. https://doi.org/10.15620/cdc:124368
19. France AM, Grant J, Kammerer JS, Navin TR. A field-validated approach using surveillance and genotyping data to estimate tuberculosis attributable to recent transmission in the United States. *Am J Epidemiol*. 2015;182(9):799–807. https://doi.org/10.1093/aje/kwv121

20. US Census Bureau. US Census Bureau geographic levels. Available at: https://www.census.gov/programs-surveys/economic-census/guidance-geographies/levels.html. Accessed May 3, 2023.

21. Jones N, Marks R, Ramirez R, Rios-Vargas M. 2020 Census illuminates racial and ethnic composition of the country. Available at: https://www.census.gov/library/stories/2021/08/improved-race-ethnicity-measures-reveal-united-states-population-much-more-multiracial.html. Accessed May 3, 2023.

22. Pew Research Center. Multiracial in America: proud, diverse and growing in numbers. 2015. Available at: https://www.pewresearch.org/social-trends/2015/06/11/multiracial-in-america. Accessed May 3, 2023.

23. Liebler CA, Porter SR, Fernandez LE, Noon JM, Ennis SR. America's churning races: race and ethnicity response changes between census 2000 and the 2010 census. *Demography.* 2017;54(1):259–284. https://doi.org/10.1007/s13524-016-0544-0

24. Connolly M, Gallagher M, Hodge F, et al. Identification in a time of invisibility for American Indians and Alaska Natives in the United States. *Stat J IAOS.* 2019;35(1):71–89. https://doi.org/10.3233/SJI-190495

COVID-19 Vaccination Rates Among North Dakota Residents Who Gave Birth Between April 1, 2021, and July 15, 2022

Olenka Aguilar, MPH, and Mary Woinarowicz, MA

Objectives. To assess COVID-19 vaccination rates among North Dakota residents who gave birth.

Methods. We used data from North Dakota Vital Records and the North Dakota Immunization Information System for North Dakota residents who gave birth between April 1, 2021, and July 15, 2022. We evaluated vaccination with 1 dose, primary series, and monovalent booster for timing before and during pregnancy and postpartum.

Results. Among North Dakota residents who gave birth, 44% received at least 1 COVID-19 vaccine, 34% received a complete primary series, and 10% received a monovalent booster dose. Among those who received a COVID-19 vaccine, the majority was vaccinated during pregnancy. Obstetrics and gynecology providers administered just 9.2% of COVID-19 vaccine doses.

Conclusions. Most persons who gave birth in North Dakota did not receive the primary series of the COVID-19 vaccine while pregnant. Providers have an opportunity to counsel their pregnant and recently pregnant patients on vaccine recommendations. (*Am J Public Health*. 2024;114(2):237–240. https://doi.org/10.2105/AJPH.2023.307500)

AJPH February 2024, Vol. 114, No. 2

The North Dakota Department of Health and Human Services (NDHHS) rolled out the first available COVID-19 vaccines in phases based on priority groups.[1] Phase 2 of the vaccine rollout began in March 2021 and made COVID-19 vaccines available to all North Dakotans older than 16 years, including pregnant persons.[2]

Pregnant persons infected with COVID-19 are at increased risk for complications and severe illness.[3] The Centers for Disease Control and Prevention, the Society for Maternal-Fetal Medicine, and the American College of Obstetricians and Gynecologists (ACOG) recommend that individuals receive COVID-19 vaccine before and during pregnancy and postpartum (6 weeks following delivery) to reduce the risk of adverse pregnancy outcomes.[3,4] ACOG encourages obstetricians and gynecologists (ob/gyn) to assess their pregnant patients' vaccination status and engage in discussions about COVID-19 vaccination.[4]

Data reported to the Vaccine Safety Datalink show pregnant persons in the United States have a lower rate of COVID-19 vaccine completion (11.1%) than do nonpregnant persons (24.9%).[5] We assessed COVID-19 vaccination rates among North Dakota residents who gave birth between April 1, 2021, and July 15, 2022.

METHODS

Using birth record data from North Dakota Vital Records, we matched a comprehensive list of persons who gave birth in North Dakota between April 1, 2021, and July 15, 2022, to immunization records from the North Dakota Immunization Information Systems (NDIIS) using first and last name and city of residence. We assessed immunization records to determine whether COVID-19 vaccine doses were administered between March 1, 2021, and August 31, 2022. The NDIIS is a confidential, population-based, information system that captures and consolidates

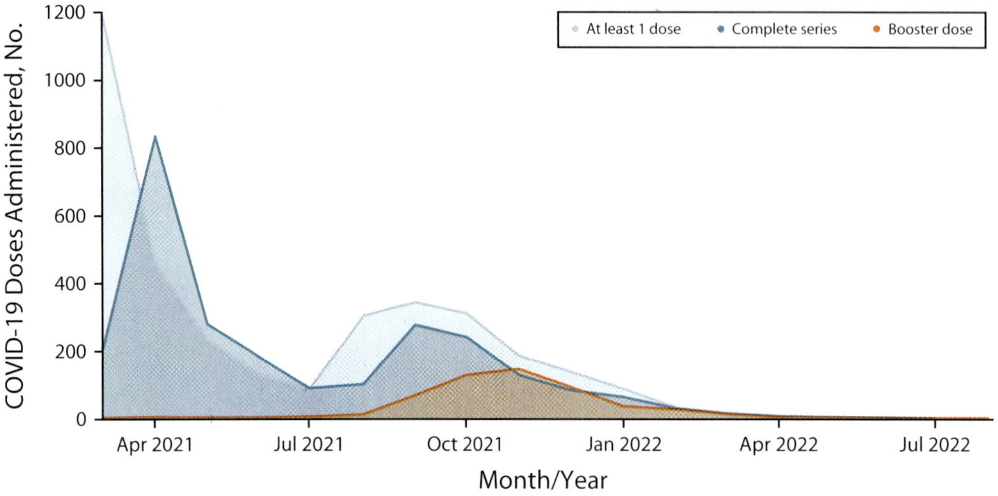

FIGURE 1— COVID-19 Doses Administered to Persons Who Gave Birth in North Dakota, by Month and Year: April 1, 2021–July 15, 2022

immunization data for all North Dakotans and includes immunization records for 100% of the state population.[6] Health care providers enrolled with the NDHHS Immunization Unit as COVID-19 vaccinators were required to report all doses administered to the NDIIS within 3 days of administration. State pharmacies and Indian Health Services vaccinators not enrolled with NDHHS reported all doses administered to the NDIIS. Vaccination data were exchanged with 2 of the 3 states that border North Dakota.

We assessed vaccination with at least 1 dose, primary series, and monovalent booster. We defined vaccination criteria as follows: 1 dose for any authorized COVID-19 vaccine, completed primary series as 2 mRNA (messenger RNA) doses or 1 Janssen dose, and monovalent booster as 3 mRNA doses or 2 Janssen doses. We assessed coverage rates by dividing the number of persons vaccinated by the number of residents who gave birth. This methodology is consistent with the established methodology for assessing COVID-19 vaccination coverage rates for the general population.[7,8]

We assessed vaccination timing by comparing babies' birthdates to the dates of vaccination and assuming 40 weeks' gestation. We determined the provider type administering the vaccine based on the facility type assigned to the COVID-19 vaccinator reporting the dose to the NDIIS.

RESULTS

We identified records for 12 503 babies born in North Dakota during the study period. NDIIS records were matched for 97% of the North Dakota residents who gave birth. Among residents who gave birth, 44%, 34%, and 10% received at least 1 dose, primary series, and a monovalent booster, respectively. Of the persons who received at least 1 dose, 65% were vaccinated during pregnancy and 35% postpartum. Of the persons who received a complete primary vaccine series, 61% completed the series during pregnancy and 39% postpartum. Of the persons who received a monovalent booster, 60% were vaccinated during pregnancy and 40% postpartum. None of the persons who gave birth during the study window received doses of the COVID-19 vaccine before pregnancy.

Among persons who gave birth and received a COVID-19 vaccine, the majority received at least 1 dose in April 2021, a primary series in May 2021, and a monovalent booster in November 2021 (Figure 1). COVID-19 vaccinators administered 10 554 doses, with the largest proportion administered by non-ob/gyn private health care providers (23.2%), local public health departments (20.9%), and hospitals (11.5%). Ob/gyn providers administered 9.2% of the COVID-19 vaccine doses.

DISCUSSION

Our results indicate vaccination peaks coinciding with the initial availability of COVID-19 vaccines for those of childbearing age, with doses peaking 2 to 3 months after recommendations and decreasing until the next recommendation (Figure 1). Peaks in COVID-19 vaccination in the US general population align with COVID-19 vaccine recommendations.[7] Given vaccine availability and the

40-week gestation period, most individuals giving birth between April 1, 2021, and July 15, 2022, were likely pregnant when the vaccine became available and did not have the opportunity for vaccination before pregnancy.

Vaccination with a primary series among North Dakota pregnant persons was lower than the general US and North Dakota populations. Among the US population and the North Dakota population, 67.9% and 56.9% of persons, respectively, were vaccinated with a primary series as of August 31, 2022.[7]

Studies report that persons who did not receive a COVID-19 vaccine were concerned about the safety of the vaccine.[9] Among unvaccinated pregnant persons, counseling from providers about COVID-19 vaccination while pregnant was found to be a predictor of vaccine acceptance.[10] Vaccine hesitancy and lack of vaccine counseling may have played a role in low vaccine uptake among pregnant persons in North Dakota, but we could not determine that impact in this evaluation.

Initially in the North Dakota COVID-19 vaccine response, vaccines were largely available only through mass vaccination events held by local public health departments and pharmacies. More than half of the unvaccinated respondents in the American COVID-19 Poll reported that their doctor's office is their preferred COVID-19 vaccination site.[11] However, we did not find an increase in doses administered by ob/gyn providers after the transition away from mass vaccination events. Vaccination setting does not seem to have had an impact on uptake of vaccine by pregnant persons.

Limitations

This study provides real-world evidence of COVID-19 vaccination practices among North Dakota residents who gave birth. Using data from North Dakota Vital Records ensured that all persons who gave birth during the study period were accounted for in the evaluation. We used a 40-week gestation to measure timing of vaccination because gestational age is not captured in the state birth record. The process of matching persons relied on exact match of names and city of residence; therefore, persons who were vaccinated but did not have a match may not have been included. Despite duplicate record-merging processes, a person may have multiple records with minor name spelling variations, making it appear like multiple individuals received a dose. Additionally, since we used data on only North Dakota residents who gave birth, the results may not be generalizable to the entire US population.

Public Health Implications

The COVID-19 vaccination rates among pregnant persons in North Dakota are low compared with the general population. Of the doses administered to pregnant persons, a majority was administered by local public health departments. We did not find an increase in doses administered by ob/gyn providers as vaccination transitioned from mass vaccination settings. These findings highlight the opportunity for ob/gyn providers to increase uptake by their pregnant patients. Ongoing monitoring of COVID-19 vaccination rates in pregnant persons and assessing why pregnant persons chose to receive or not to receive the COVID-19 is critical to understanding vaccine uptake in this population. AJPH

ABOUT THE AUTHORS

Olenka Aguilar is with the CDC Foundation, Atlanta, GA. Mary Woinarowicz is with the North Dakota Department of Health and Human Services, Bismarck.

CORRESPONDENCE

Correspondence should be sent to Mary Woinarowicz, NDIIS Manager, North Dakota Department of Health, 600 E Boulevard Ave, Dept 301, Bismarck, ND 58505-0200 (e-mail: mary.woinarowicz@nd.gov). Reprints can be ordered at http://www.ajph.org by clicking the "Reprints" link.

PUBLICATION INFORMATION

Full Citation: Aguilar O, Woinarowicz M. COVID-19 vaccination rates among North Dakota residents who gave birth between April 1, 2021, and July 15, 2022. *Am J Public Health*. 2024;114(2): 237–240.

Acceptance Date: October 13, 2023.

DOI: https://doi.org/10.2105/AJPH.2023.307500

CONTRIBUTORS

O. Aguilar designed the evaluation project, conducted the data analysis, and was the primary author on the article. M. Woinarowicz provided subject matter expertise and input on immunizations, North Dakota Immunization Information System data, and data analysis and provided oversight and input on the article.

ACKNOWLEDGMENTS

This project was supported by the Centers for Disease Control and Prevention (CDC) of the US Department of Health and Human Services (HHS) as part of the cooperative agreement funding opportunity IP19-1901.

Note. The findings and conclusions in this article are those of the authors and do not necessarily represent the official position of the North Dakota Department of Health and Human Services, the CDC, the HHS, or the US government.

CONFLICTS OF INTEREST

The authors have no potential or actual conflicts of interest from funding or affiliation-related activities.

HUMAN PARTICIPANT PROTECTION

The authors received a waiver of institutional review board (IRB) approval from the North Dakota Department of Health and Human Services Public Health Division IRB because evaluation of immunization coverage rates among the North Dakota population is standard public health practice.

REFERENCES

1. North Dakota Department of Health. Phases for COVID-19 vaccine. March 8, 2021. Available at: https://www.hhs.nd.gov/sites/www/files/documents/DOH%20Legacy/COVID-19_Vaccine_Prioritization_Phase_1A-C.pdf. Accessed March 23, 2022.
2. State of North Dakota. Department of Health announces COVID-19 vaccine will be available to

the general public on March 29. March 19, 2021. Available at: https://ndresponse.gov/news/department-health-announces-covid-19-vaccine-will-be-available-general-public-march-29. Accessed March 23, 2022.

3. Centers for Disease Control and Prevention. Pregnant and recently pregnant people. October 25, 2022. Available at: https://www.cdc.gov/coronavirus/2019-ncov/need-extra-precautions/pregnant-people.html#print. Accessed March 23, 2022.
4. American College of Obstetricians and Gynecologists. COVID-19 vaccination considerations for obstetric–gynecologic care. March 2, 2022. Available at: https://www.acog.org/clinical/clinical-guidance/practice-advisory/articles/2020/12/covid-19-vaccination-considerations-for-obstetric-gynecologic-care. Accessed March 25, 2022.
5. Centers for Disease Control and Prevention. COVID-19 vaccination coverage among adults—United States, December 14, 2020–May 22, 2021. *MMWR Morb Mortal Wkly Rep.* 2021;70(25):922–927. https://doi.org/10.15585/mmwr.mm7025e1
6. Centers for Disease Control and Prevention. About immunization information systems. June 7, 2019. Available at: https://www.cdc.gov/vaccines/programs/iis/about.html. Accessed July 5, 2022.
7. Centers for Disease Control and Prevention. COVID data tracker. May 11, 2023. Available at: https://covid.cdc.gov/covid-data-tracker/#vaccination-trends. Accessed January 23, 2023.
8. Centers for Disease Control and Prevention. Data definitions for COVID-19 vaccinations in the United States. January 20, 2023. Available at: https://www.cdc.gov/coronavirus/2019-ncov/vaccines/reporting-vaccinations.html. Accessed January 23, 2023.
9. Levy AT, Singh S, Riley LE, Prabhu M. Acceptance of COVID-19 vaccination in pregnancy: a survey study. *Am J Obstet Gynecol MFM*. 2021;3(5):100399. https://doi.org/10.1016/j.ajogmf.2021.100399
10. Huddleston HG, Jaswa EG, Lindquist KJ, et al. COVID-19 vaccination patterns and attitudes among American pregnant individuals. *Am J Obstet Gynecol MFM*. 2022;4(1):100507. https://doi.org/10.1016/j.ajogmf.2021.100507
11. African American Research Collaborative. American COVID-19 vaccine poll. 2021. Available at: https://covidvaccinepoll.com/app/aarc/covid-19-vaccine-messaging/#. Accessed June 14, 2022.

Patient Acceptability of Telehealth Medication Abortion Care in the United States, 2021–2022: A Cohort Study

Leah R. Koenig, MSPH, Jennifer Ko, MLIS, Ena Suseth Valladares, MPH, Francine M. Coeytaux, MPH, Elisa Wells, MPH, Courtney R. Lyles, PhD, and Ushma D. Upadhyay, PhD, MPH

See also Munson and Hall, p. 152.

Objectives. Despite the recent expansion of direct-to-patient telehealth abortion care in the United States, patient experiences with the service are not well understood.

Methods. We described care experiences of 1600 telehealth abortion patients in 2021 to 2022 and used logistic regression to explore differences by race or ethnicity and between synchronous (phone or video) and asynchronous (secure messaging) telehealth abortion care.

Results. Most patients trusted the provider (98%), felt telehealth was the right decision (96%), felt cared for (92%), and were very satisfied (89%). Patients most commonly cited privacy (76%), timeliness (74%), and staying at home (71%) as benefits. The most commonly reported drawback was initial uncertainty about whether the service was legitimate (38%). Asian patients were less likely to be very satisfied than White patients (79% vs 90%; $P = .008$). Acceptability was high for both synchronous and asynchronous care.

Conclusions. Telehealth abortion care is highly acceptable, and benefits include privacy and expediency.

Public Health Implications. Telehealth abortion can expand abortion access in an increasingly restricted landscape while maintaining patient-centered care. (*Am J Public Health*. 2024;114(2):241–250. https://doi.org/10.2105/AJPH.2023.307437)

AJPH February 2024, Vol. 114, No. 2

In the wake of the June 2022 *Dobbs v Jackson* Supreme Court decision that allowed states to ban abortion, telehealth medication abortion has played a vital role in abortion provision and access in the United States. Telehealth can help mitigate surges in demand for abortion care in states where it remains legal.[1,2] For patients in states with abortion bans, telehealth services can also increase abortion access through methods like mail forwarding and mailing medications to a postal address or post office box in neighboring states over the border, minimizing the amount of travel required.

Medication abortion has emerged as the leading abortion method both within[3] and outside of[4] the health care system in the United States in recent years. Concurrently, there has been a rise in medication abortion provided via telehealth, facilitated by regulatory changes that allowed abortion medications to be mailed beginning in the COVID-19 pandemic.[5] Before the pandemic, telehealth abortion models were primarily "site-to-site," requiring patients to travel to abortion clinics, where they received ultrasonography and other in-person tests and then remotely consulted with a clinician who was at another location.[6,7]

Direct-to-patient telehealth abortion care first became widely available in the United States in 2020 and has been found to be safe and effective.[8–10] Since then, virtual clinics—online-only abortion providers—began providing this model of telehealth abortion care in states where it is legally permitted.[11–13] Patients are screened for eligibility remotely by a clinician, receiving an ultrasound only if desired or medically indicated, and subsequently receive medications from a mail-order pharmacy.[14] In all medication abortion care models, patients typically take the medications, pass the pregnancy, and complete follow-up at home.[15] Patient–provider communication is either entirely over secure text messaging (asynchronous care) or with a videoconference or phone call (synchronous care).[16]

As of November 2023, telehealth for abortion was legally permitted in 24 states and Washington, DC (Figure A, available as a supplement to the online version of this article at https://ajph.org).[17] Between April 2022 and June 2023, the number of abortions provided by virtual clinics nearly doubled, accounting for almost 1 in 10 US abortions by June 2023.[2]

Despite the critical role that telehealth plays in maintaining access to abortion across an increasingly restricted landscape, the acceptability of direct-to-patient telehealth for abortion in the United States is not well understood. Evidence from the TelAbortion study has demonstrated US patients' positive experiences with synchronous telehealth abortion care within a clinical study.[9,18–20] No studies have examined differences in patient experiences between synchronous and asynchronous care. Telehealth medication abortion care models are less medicalized compared with in-clinic care, and differences in experiences by patient sociodemographic characteristics have not been documented. As ongoing legal cases threaten to curtail access to telehealth abortion, it is critical to understand how patients experience these models of care. Therefore, we aimed to explore the real-world acceptability of novel direct-to-patient abortion services provided by US virtual clinics and to examine differences in abortion care experiences between synchronous and asynchronous models and patient sociodemographic characteristics.

METHODS

We used data from the California Home Abortion by Telehealth (CHAT) Study, which evaluates the safety, effectiveness, and acceptability of telehealth abortion care provided by 3 United States–based virtual clinics. The CHAT Study began in California and increased in scope as virtual clinics expanded to provide care in 20 states and Washington, DC. The study collected electronic clinical data from all abortions provided by the participating clinics for a defined period between April 2021 and January 2022. During clinic intake, patients consented to share anonymized data with our research team. Patients approved for care between June 2021 and January 2022 were also invited to participate in a series of 3 surveys: 1 at abortion intake, another in the week after intake, and a final survey 4 weeks after intake. The baseline survey assessed patient sociodemographic characteristics and initial reasons for choosing telehealth. The first follow-up survey assessed medication administration and additional medical care received. The final survey assessed additional medical care received and experiences with the telehealth model including open-ended and closed-ended questions. Surveys were administered until all 3 surveys were completed by approximately 400 participants from each clinic. Participants received $50 as remuneration after the completion of all 3 surveys.

One clinic used synchronous communication with a phone or video call to screen patients for eligibility. The other 2 screened patients through asynchronous communication, which involved an online consultation form and subsequent communication via secure written messages. One of the clinics that screened patients through asynchronous communication by default also offered the option to request a synchronous intake appointment. Abortion costs from the 3 virtual clinics ranged from $199 to $239. During the study period, virtual clinics did not accept health insurance; however, each clinic offered financial assistance for the cost of the abortion via abortion funds.

Measures

We used several indicators of patient acceptability as the main outcome measures (Table A, available as a supplement to the online version of this article at https://ajph.org). We examined participants' reasons for choosing telehealth reported in the baseline survey; participants could select all reasons that applied. The remaining outcome measures were asked in the 4-week follow-up survey. We assessed overall satisfaction, with Likert scale response options categorized into "very satisfied" versus other responses. We assessed whether participants could trust the virtual clinic with their care, whether they felt cared for throughout the abortion process, and whether telehealth was the right decision for them using individual dichotomous items ("yes" vs "no" or "don't know"). Open-ended questions modeled the closed-ended items, assessing reasons for choosing telehealth, benefits of telehealth abortion, why they did or did not feel cared for, and how they felt like they could or could not trust the virtual clinic.

The baseline survey asked participants to identify the benefits and drawbacks of the telehealth abortion model in 2 select-all-that-apply items, with the option to write in other responses. Other responses were coded into closed-ended responses, the most common of which are represented in the results.

Our primary key predictor was whether patient acceptability outcomes differed between those who received synchronous and asynchronous abortion care. Our secondary key predictor was the participant's race or ethnicity. Covariates included categorized measures of participant age at abortion intake, pregnancy duration on the day of abortion intake, education level, and health insurance coverage. We included binary measures reflecting experiences of food insecurity in the past month, previous medication abortion, whether the participant was born outside of the United States, and whether their zip code corresponded to an urban, or a suburban or rural area.

Statistical Analysis

We reported sample characteristics using descriptive statistics and used the χ^2 and Fisher exact test to examine differences between the groups that received synchronous and asynchronous care. We used multivariable logistic regression to examine associations between participant and abortion model characteristics, and each patient acceptability indicator. Patient age (< 25 years; 25–29 years; 30–34 years; ≥ 35 years), pregnancy duration (< 35 days; 35–49 days; ≥ 50 days), and race or ethnicity categories (White; Black; Hispanic or Latinx; Asian, Native Hawaiian, or Pacific Islander; American Indian or Alaska Native, Middle Eastern or North African, or multiracial) were collapsed in the regression analyses to facilitate model convergence. We used predictive margins to calculate adjusted rates of each patient acceptability indicator.

Open-Text Responses

To illustrate meaning and provide context for the quantitative results, we purposively selected from the open-ended survey responses. L. R. K. and U. D. U. identified candidate quotes that corresponded to each patient acceptability indicator, among which L. R. K. selected final quotes for inclusion.

RESULTS

Originally, 1632 participants enrolled in the longitudinal surveys (32% of invited patients). Among those, we excluded 32 participants who took neither mifepristone nor misoprostol, resulting in an initial sample of 1600 survey participants in 20 states and Washington, DC. Ultimately, 1312 (82%) completed the 4-week follow-up survey.

We described sample characteristics in Table 1. At abortion intake, mean participant age was 29 years and mean pregnancy duration was 40 days (< 7 weeks). Across the sample, 53% identified as White; 14% as multiple races or ethnicities; 13% as Hispanic or Latinx; 9% as Black; 6% as Asian, Native Hawaiian, or Pacific Islander; 1% as American Indian, Native American, or Alaska Native; and 1% as Middle Eastern or North African. Nearly half (42%) had completed college or more education, and 21% experienced running out of food in the past month. Most (89%) participants were born in the United States and resided in urban areas (91%). More than half (56%) resided in the US West, 20% in the Northeast, and smaller proportions in the Midwest (12%) and South (12%). One third (29%) had a previous medication abortion and 59% had private health insurance. One third (31%) had a video or phone call during abortion intake (synchronous care). At the clinic that provided asynchronous care but offered the option to request synchronous care, 1% received synchronous care.

Motivations for and Benefits of Telehealth

We examined participants' reasons for choosing telehealth at baseline (Figure 1). The most common reasons for choosing telehealth were feeling more comfortable at home (75%) and privacy (59%). Participants explained the importance of these features in open-ended responses:

> I felt more comfortable and less anxious about the whole process from being able to be home. I really appreciate having the opportunity to be in the comfort of my own home for the abortion and with my spouse for the entire duration and not in a cold room with strangers to have an uncomfortable procedure. –Age 26 years, Georgia, synchronous care

More than half (58%) identified lower costs relative to in-clinic care as a reason for using telehealth, a theme that participants expanded on in open-ended responses:

> I couldn't afford a surgical or medical abortion from the clinic. [Telehealth care] is half the price of abortions where I live. –Age 21 years, Oregon, synchronous care

More than half (55%) of respondents endorsed a desire to have the abortion

TABLE 1— Characteristics of the Sample: United States, 2021–2022

Characteristic	Overall (n = 1600), No. (%)	Synchronous (n = 503), No. (%)	Asynchronous (n = 1097), No. (%)	P
Patient age at abortion intake, y				.07
16–17	8 (< 1)	0 (0)	8 (1)	
18–19	67 (4)	14 (3)	53 (5)	
20–24	381 (24)	111 (22)	270 (25)	
25–29	418 (26)	138 (27)	280 (26)	
30–34	405 (25)	140 (28)	265 (24)	
≥ 35	321 (20)	100 (20)	221 (20)	
Pregnancy duration at abortion intake, d				< .001
< 35	448 (28)	161 (32)	287 (26)	
35–49	885 (55)	294 (58)	591 (54)	
50–62	229 (14)	46 (9)	183 (17)	
≥ 63	38 (2)	2 (< 1)	36 (3)	
Race or ethnicity				< .001
Non-Hispanic White	841 (53)	285 (57)	556 (51)	
Non-Hispanic Black or African American	148 (9)	68 (14)	80 (7)	
Hispanic or Latinx	203 (13)	46 (9)	157 (14)	
American Indian, Alaska Native, Middle Eastern, North African, or multiracial	237 (15)	60 (12)	177 (16)	
Asian, Native Hawaiian, or Pacific Islander	105 (7)	19 (4)	86 (8)	
Unknown	66 (4)	25 (5)	41 (4)	
Food did not last, last month				< .001
No	1207 (75)	393 (78)	814 (74)	
Yes	340 (21)	82 (16)	258 (24)	
Unknown	53 (3)	28 (6)	25 (2)	
Previous medication abortion				.61
No	1136 (71)	349 (69)	787 (72)	
Yes	457 (29)	152 (30)	305 (28)	
Unknown	7 (< 1)	2 (< 1)	5 (< 1)	
US region				< .001
West	896 (56)	177 (35)	719 (66)	
Northeast	313 (20)	99 (20)	214 (20)	
South	195 (12)	181 (36)	14 (1)	
Midwest	196 (12)	46 (9)	150 (14)	
Highest level of education achieved				< .001
High school or less	274 (17)	62 (12)	212 (19)	
Some college or technical school	659 (41)	200 (40)	459 (42)	
Completed 4-y degree or more	667 (42)	241 (48)	426 (39)	
Health insurance coverage				.019
Private insurance	941 (59)	315 (63)	626 (57)	
No insurance	317 (20)	83 (17)	234 (21)	
Medicaid	293 (18)	96 (19)	197 (18)	
Unknown	49 (3)	9 (2)	40 (4)	
Nativity				< .001
Born in the United States	1430 (89)	435 (86)	995 (91)	

Continued

TABLE 1— Continued

Characteristic	Overall (n = 1600), No. (%)	Synchronous (n = 503), No. (%)	Asynchronous (n = 1097), No. (%)	P
Born outside the United States	138 (9)	44 (9)	94 (9)	
Unknown	32 (2)	24 (5)	8 (1)	
Residence				.59
Suburban or rural	146 (9)	43 (9)	103 (9)	
Urban	1454 (91)	460 (91)	994 (91)	
Completion of 4-wk follow-up survey				< .001
Did not complete survey	288 (18)	27 (5)	261 (24)	
Completed survey	1312 (82)	476 (95)	836 (76)	

Note. The sample size was 1600.

as soon as possible, and many cited long waiting times at abortion clinics as a reason for choosing telehealth in open-ended fields:

> The biggest thing was time. [Clinics were] booked out for weeks, and I didn't want to wait weeks. –Age 32 years, Oregon, synchronous care

Meanwhile, 44% were motivated to use telehealth because it allowed them to take care of their own treatment. One participant explained,

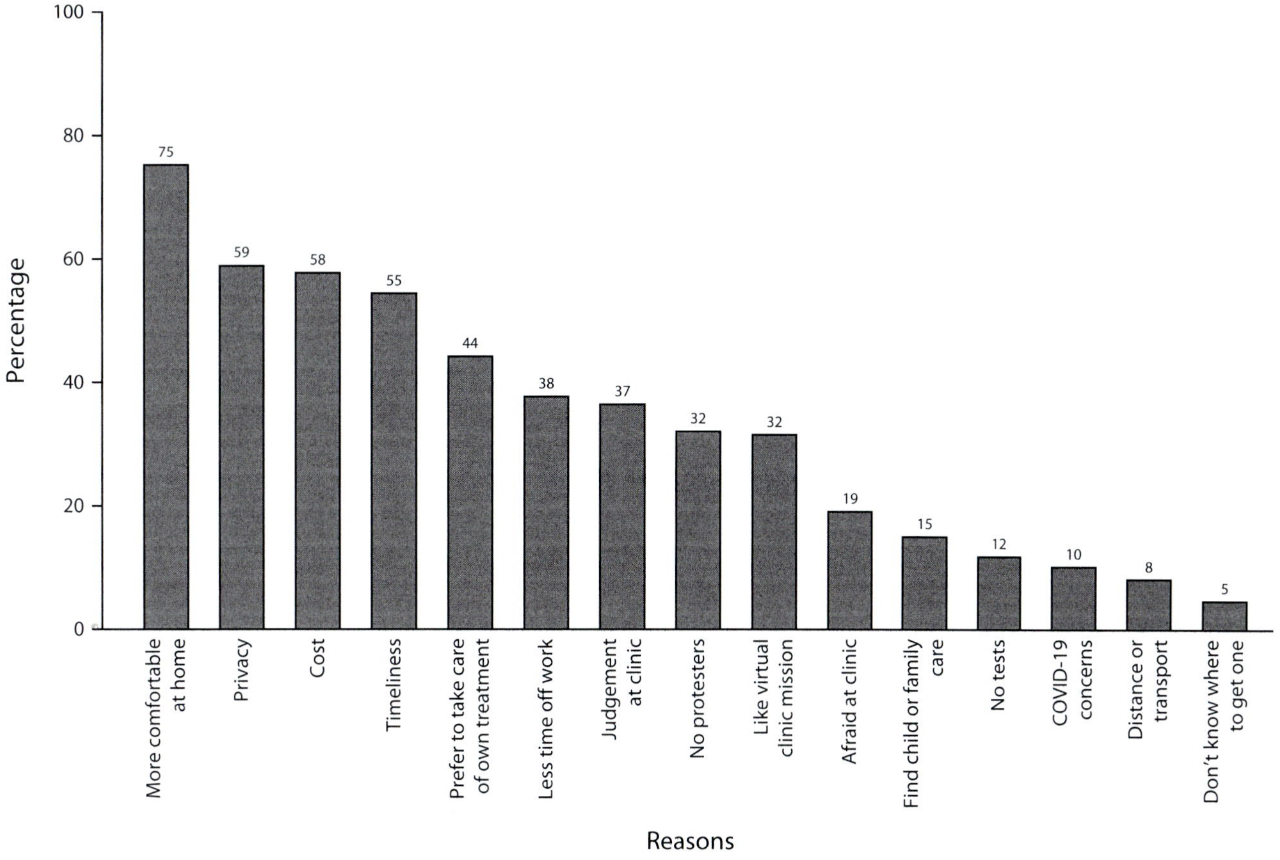

FIGURE 1— Reasons for Choosing Telehealth: United States, 2021–2022

Note. The sample size was 1600.

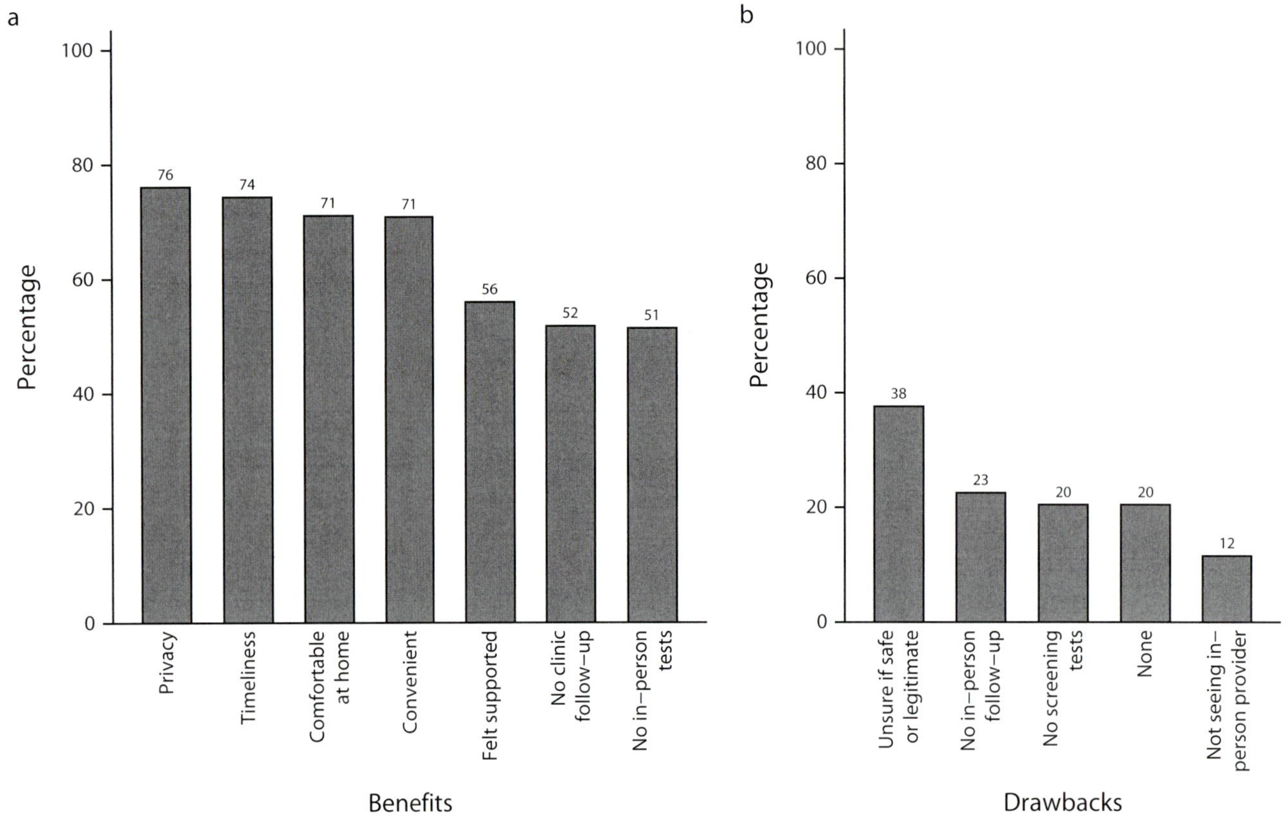

FIGURE 2— Telehealth Abortion (a) Benefits and (b) Drawbacks: United States, 2021–2022

Note. The sample size was 1312.

> I appreciate this experience of having the autonomy to be able to manage my own care with adequate support from a nurse practitioner. –Age 32 years, Illinois, asynchronous care

Similarly, another participant wrote,

> I felt more safe or secure, more empowered doing it my own way. –Age 26 years, California, asynchronous care

At the 4-week follow-up survey, the most common benefits of telehealth that participants cited were privacy (76%), expediency (74%), being more comfortable at home (71%), and convenience (71%; Figure 2). Overall, 56% of participants endorsed feeling supported as a benefit, and half cited not needing to go to the clinic for in-person screening tests (51%) or for follow-up (52%). One participant described their preference to have their abortion without ultrasound:

> At a stressful time, I don't want to be subjected to a vaginal ultrasound and blood work. If I know when I got pregnant, I don't need an ultrasound. –Age 36 years, Illinois, asynchronous care

Drawbacks of Telehealth

When asked about the drawbacks of telehealth, the most common response was uncertainty about whether the service was safe or legitimate (38%). Some participants described deciding to place their trust in the virtual clinic as a leap of faith:

> Not having any other option made me trust the service. There were times I doubted it could possibly be this easy or straightforward without there being some horrible catch. –Age 36 years, New Jersey, synchronous care

Overall, 20% reported no drawbacks. About one fifth cited not having screening (20%) and follow-up (23%) tests as drawbacks of their telehealth abortion experience. One participant stated,

> I would have liked confirmation that it was complete via ultrasound. –Age 29 years, New York, asynchronous care

TABLE 2— Associations Between Patient and Abortion Characteristic and Acceptability Indicators: United States, 2021–2022

	Very Satisfied, PPR (95% CI)	Right Decision, PPR (95% CI)	Trust Provider, PPR (95% CI)	Cared for, PPR (95% CI)
Overall	89.7 (88.0, 91.4)	95.6 (94.4, 96.7)	98.0 (97.1, 98.8)	91.9 (90.4, 93.4)
Model of care				
Synchronous (n = 476; Ref)	90.4 (87.7, 93.2)	97.1 (95.6, 98.6)	97.3 (95.8, 98.8)	88.5 (85.5, 91.4)
Asynchronous (n = 836)	88.7 (86.5, 90.9)	94.7 (93.1, 96.2)	98.3 (97.5, 99.2)	93.4 (91.7, 95.1)**
Race or ethnicity				
Non-Hispanic White (n = 689; Ref)	89.5 (87.2, 91.8)	95.4 (93.7, 97.0)	97.9 (96.7, 99.1)	92.7 (90.7, 94.6)
Non-Hispanic Black or African American (n = 121)	91.4 (86.3, 96.5)	95.1 (91.3, 99.0)	97.9 (95.4, 100.0)	88.6 (83.0, 94.3)
Hispanic or Latinx[a] (n = 166)	90.7 (86.1, 95.2)	97.3 (94.9, 99.7)	98.8 (97.5, 100.0)	95.1 (91.5, 98.7)
American Indian, Alaska Native, Middle Eastern, North African, or multiracial (n = 194)	91.1 (87.2, 95.0)	97.1 (94.8, 99.4)	96.8 (94.3, 99.3)	89.6 (85.4, 93.9)
Asian, Native Hawaiian, or Pacific Islander[a] (n = 87)	78.5 (69.0, 87.9)**	91.5 (85.4, 97.7)	98.8 (97.5, 100.0)	87.7 (79.9, 95.6)

Note. CI = confidence interval; PPR = predicted prevalence rate. The sample size was n = 1312. Estimates are PPRs that draw from marginal estimates of multivariable logistic regression models. *P* values compare each category to the reference group in the multivariable logistic regression models. Multivariable models are adjusted for synchronous versus asynchronous care, patient age at abortion intake, pregnancy duration at abortion intake, food insecurity in the past month, race or ethnicity, previous medication abortion, education level, health insurance coverage, US nativity, and urban residence.

[a]Variable for race or ethnicity combined Hispanic or Latinx with Asian, Native Hawaiian, or Pacific Islander for the "trust provider" model.
*$P < .05$; **$P < .01$; ***$P < .001$.

A smaller proportion (12%) listed not seeing a provider in person as a drawback of the telehealth model. In the open-ended responses, some participants also described being unable to reach the virtual clinic at times:

> I took my pills on the weekend, so I had nobody to contact, which was unfortunate because I really wasn't sure if the severity of what I was experiencing was normal. –Age 24 years, California, asynchronous care

Overall Rates of Acceptability Indicators

We next examined the adjusted proportion of participants who reported each of the 4 patient acceptability indicators of interest: trust, right decision, cared for, and satisfied (Table 2). Overall, 98% trusted the virtual clinic, 96% felt telehealth was the right decision, 92% felt cared for, and 90% of participants were very satisfied with the telehealth model of care. Full regression output is presented in Table B (available as a supplement to the online version of this article at https://ajph.org).

Differences in Patient Acceptability by Participant Characteristics

Finally, we assessed differences in adjusted prevalence rates of each patient acceptability indicator by participant characteristics (Table 2). Asian, Native Hawaiian, and Pacific Islander participants were less likely than White participants to be very satisfied (79% vs 90%; $P = .008$). Similar proportions of patients who received synchronous and asynchronous care were very satisfied, felt telehealth was the right decision, and felt cared for by the telehealth provider. However, participants who had asynchronous care were slightly more likely to feel cared for (93% vs 89%; $P = .004$).

In the open-ended responses, we found that some participants stated clear preferences for synchronous care, while others clearly preferred asynchronous care. One participant explained their preference for asynchronous care because it facilitated anonymity:

> Everything was very professional and never pressed for any information. There was no pressure to do an appointment showing who I was. Privacy was well respected, and the ball was in my court to decide how much care I wish to receive (ex. seeing the doctor or nurse). –Age 29 years, California, asynchronous care

However, some participants who received asynchronous care described how asynchronous communication could feel impersonal. One participant wrote,

> Since I talked to a nurse through chat, it didn't feel personable, and I wasn't sure if I was getting an automated message or if I was chatting with an actual person. –Age 27 years, California, asynchronous care

Another participant described how their synchronous care facilitated trust in the virtual clinic, despite initial reluctance about a video call:

> It was the video call! It proved it was a real service and that it was their focus at [the virtual clinic]. As much as I didn't want to do a video call, it helped solidify the legitimacy of the service. –Age 41 years, California, asynchronous care

One participant explained how being offered options for both synchronous and asynchronous services was important to their care:

> I knew it was legitimate because they were considering all the right things: the 24/7 hotline, video calls if we want but also that they aren't necessary. You can make it into the right abortion care for you. I personally didn't make any calls or message much, but I trust the service because I know I can get whatever help I need. –Age 23 years, Washington, asynchronous care

Another participant stated,

> They gave me a number to call if I needed, texted multiple times, and always said to text (which I love because I hate talking on the phone), or to call if I needed anything or had questions. –Age 43 years, California, asynchronous care

DISCUSSION

In this study, we found high acceptability of telehealth for abortion, whether it involved synchronous or asynchronous services. Nearly all participants were very satisfied with telehealth abortion. Telehealth abortion care is a new service and, thus, it was previously unknown whether this less medicalized model that eliminates in-person patient–provider interaction would negatively impact patient acceptability. Of course, telehealth abortion care is not for everyone, including individuals who are seeking abortion care later in pregnancy, those who prefer procedural abortions, and those who prefer to have screening and follow-up tests as a part of their medication abortion care. Thus, while access to in-person abortion care remains critical, this study indicates that telehealth is an important addition to the abortion landscape and offers substantial benefits over in-person care for some patients.

The most common reason for choosing telehealth was that patients felt more comfortable at home. Most patients also reported choosing telehealth for greater privacy, lower cost, expediency, and more agency in managing their abortion care. Thus, telehealth abortion appears to help mitigate some barriers patients face in accessing care from an abortion clinic. Beyond its role in increasing access to abortion care and addressing the surges abortion facilities face as patients travel in wake of *Dobbs*, telehealth can promote patient-centered care for some people seeking an abortion.[18,21]

We found few differences in acceptability between synchronous or asynchronous telehealth abortion care: patients were equally likely to be highly satisfied, trust the virtual clinic, and feel telehealth was the right decision. These findings suggest that both synchronous and asynchronous models are highly acceptable to patients. We found slightly higher rates of feeling cared for among participants who received asynchronous services. When patients from one clinic were offered asynchronous telehealth abortion services by default with an additional option for synchronous communication, almost no patients opted for synchronous care. While our results were largely similar for the 2 models, there may be different benefits and drawbacks of synchronous and asynchronous care with implications for providers and administrators. Services without real-time communication are presumed to feel less personable, but messaging can facilitate more frequent and responsive communication, which may contribute to patients feeling cared for. In addition, asynchronous models can require less time to provide, making them more cost-effective.[22,23] Our results demonstrate that asynchronous services can be provided while maintaining high levels of patient acceptability.

Nearly 40% of the sample was initially uncertain whether the virtual clinic services were safe or legitimate. At the time of the study, telehealth abortion services and virtual clinics were newly available within the formal US health care system. We expect that skepticism about legitimacy will decrease over time as public awareness about the safety and effectiveness of telehealth abortion increases. While these data draw from a time when interest in telehealth was very high because of the COVID-19 pandemic, use of telehealth abortion has continued to expand as barriers to access abortion care mount.[2]

We found few differences in acceptability of telehealth abortion care by race or ethnicity in this sample, apart from finding lower rates of satisfaction among Asian versus White participants. Asian Americans are underrepresented among abortion patients, which could contribute to stigma and help to explain these findings.[24] Research has found lower levels of broader telehealth adoption among Asian individuals despite high levels of digital connectedness, which may be explained by discrimination in medical settings.[25]

Limitations

This analysis has several limitations. First, all participants self-selected into telehealth care. Participants in our study were disproportionately older, White, and more financially secure than the national population of abortion patients,[24] although our sample may be more representative of the 24 states where telehealth abortion is legal. In addition, virtual clinic abortion services were available only in English and required a credit or debit card. These factors may limit the generalizability of our findings, leading us to find higher acceptability than we would have seen if patients had been more representative of the general abortion patient population. While our follow-up rate was high compared with other medication abortion studies, 18% of the sample was lost to follow-up, which may have introduced selection bias. This could have overestimated patient acceptability if those less satisfied dropped out of the study at higher rates or underestimated acceptability if participants for whom privacy was very important were more likely to be lost to follow-up. Finally, our study had limited variation in synchronous and asynchronous care among the 3 included clinics and an insufficient number of clusters to calculate clustered standard errors within each virtual clinic. Therefore, our study may have overestimated differences in acceptability of care if the observed differences between synchronous and asynchronous are truly attributable to differences in acceptability across the virtual clinics. However, each virtual clinic had multiple clinicians, bolstering the validity of the differences we detected.

Public Health Implications

In a post-Roe world, telehealth is taking on a greater role in the US abortion care landscape. Therefore, medication abortion, and telehealth medication abortion specifically, has become a focus of abortion restrictions. The high patient satisfaction with telehealth abortion found in this study combined with documentation of the safety and effectiveness of this service delivery modality[8,26] supports its continued availability.

Although this study found very high patient satisfaction with telehealth abortion, it is critical to understand abortion service delivery preferences and lower levels of acceptability among Asian patients. Our data suggest that telehealth is disproportionately accessible to patient populations who face fewer barriers to in-clinic abortion care. Policy and service changes that facilitate patients' use of Medicaid and insurance to pay for the abortion, offer services in multiple languages, and increase minors' access to care are critical to ensuring a range of accessible and acceptable telehealth abortion models.[21] Given increasing barriers to abortion across the United States, it is essential to further develop innovative models of care and ensure that all people who need abortion care will have access to a service delivery model that is right for them. AJPH

ABOUT THE AUTHORS

Leah R. Koenig, Jennifer Ko, and Ushma D. Upadhyay are with Advancing New Standards in Reproductive Health, Department of Obstetrics, Gynecology and Reproductive Sciences, University of California, San Francisco, Oakland. Ena Suseth Valladares is with California Latinas for Reproductive Justice, Los Angeles. Francine M. Coeytaux and Elisa Wells are with Plan C. Courtney R. Lyles is with the Department of Epidemiology and Biostatistics, University of California, San Francisco.

CORRESPONDENCE

Correspondence should be sent to Ushma D. Upadhyay, PhD, MPH, Advancing New Standards in Reproductive Health, University of California, San Francisco, 1330 Broadway, Suite 1100, Oakland, CA 94612 (e-mail: ushma.upadhyay@ucsf.edu). Reprints can be ordered at https://ajph.org by clicking the "Reprints" link.

PUBLICATION INFORMATION

Full Citation: Koenig LR, Ko J, Valladares ES, et al. Patient acceptability of telehealth medication abortion care in the United States, 2021–2022: a cohort study. *Am J Public Health*. 2024;114(2): 241–250.

Acceptance Date: August 28, 2023.

DOI: https://doi.org/10.2105/AJPH.2023.307437

CONTRIBUTORS

L. R. Koenig conceptualized the analysis, conducted the data analysis, drafted the article, interpreted the data, and coordinated subsequent revisions. J. Ko provided administrative support for the study, interpreted the data, reviewed drafts of the article, and revised the article. E. S. Valladares, F. M. Coeytaux, E. Wells, and C. R. Lyles interpreted the data, reviewed drafts of the article, and provided substantive input on its content. U. D. Upadhyay obtained funding, supervised data analysis, drafted the article, interpreted the data, and revised the article.

ACKNOWLEDGMENTS

This research was supported by the BaSe Family Fund, the Erik E. and Edith H. Bergstrom Foundation, the Lisa and Douglas Goldman Fund, the Isabel Allende Foundation, Jess Jacobs, the Kahle/Austin Foundation, and Preston-Werner Ventures. L. R. Koenig was funded in part by a training grant from the National Institute on Minority Health and Health Disparities of the National Institutes of Health under award T32MD015070 and the National Institute of Child Health and Human Development under award F31HD111277 for the duration of the study. C. R. Lyles was supported by a University of California San Francisco–Genentech Mid-Career Development Award.

The authors appreciate contributions to data collection and management and other input on the California Home Abortion by Telehealth Study from Linda Shin, Kelly Song, Andréa Becker, and Lisa Peters. We thank Cindy Adam, Mark Adam, Kate Baron, Stephanie Bussmann, Leah Coplon, Lauren Dubey, Lindsay DuBois, Kiki Freedman, Gaby Izarra, Jamie Phifer, and Aisha Wagner for supporting data acquisition.

Note. The funders had no role in the study design, data collection and analysis, writing of the report, or the decision to submit the article for publication.

CONFLICTS OF INTEREST

C. R. Lyles receives contract funding from AppliedVR, InquisitHealth, and Somnology and was a visiting researcher at Google in 2022–2023.

HUMAN PARTICIPANT PROTECTION

The study was approved by the University of California, San Francisco's institutional review board (20-32951).

REFERENCES

1. Aiken AR, Upadhyay UD. The future of medication abortion in a post-Roe world. *BMJ*. 2022; 337:o1393. https://doi.org/10.1136/bmj.o1393
2. #WeCount Report April 2022 to June 2023 Findings. Denver, CO: Society of Family Planning; October, 2023. https://doi.org/10.46621/218569qkgmbl
3. Jones R, Nash E, Cross L, Philbin J, Kirstein M. Medication abortion now accounts for more than half of all US abortions. New York, NY: Guttmacher Institute; 2022.
4. Aiken ARA, Starling JE, van der Wal A, et al. Demand for self-managed medication abortion through an online telemedicine service in the United States. *Am J Public Health*. 2020;110(1): 90–97. https://doi.org/10.2105/AJPH.2019.305369
5. Cavazzoni P. Response letter from FDA CDER to American Association of Pro-Life Obstetricians and Gynecologists and American College of Pediatricians. December 17, 2021. Available at: https://www.regulations.gov/document/FDA-2019-P-1534-0016. Accessed February 10, 2023.
6. Grossman DA, Grindlay K, Buchacker T, Potter JE, Schmertmann CP. Changes in service delivery patterns after introduction of telemedicine provision of medical abortion in Iowa. *Am J Public Health*. 2013;103(1):73–78. https://doi.org/10.2105/AJPH.2012.301097
7. Seymour JW, Thompson TA, Milechin D, Wise LA, Rudolph AE. Potential impact of telemedicine for medication abortion policy and programming changes on abortion accessibility in the United States. *Am J Public Health*. 2022;112(8):1202–1211. https://doi.org/10.2105/AJPH.2022.306876
8. Upadhyay UD, Koenig LR, Meckstroth KR. Safety and efficacy of telehealth medication abortions in the US during the COVID-19 pandemic. *JAMA Netw Open*. 2021;4(8):e2122320. https://doi.org/10.1001/jamanetworkopen.2021.22320
9. Anger HA, Raymond EG, Grant M, et al. Clinical and service delivery implications of omitting ultrasound before medication abortion provided via direct-to-patient telemedicine and mail in the US *Contraception*. 2021;104(6):659–665. https://doi.org/10.1016/j.contraception.2021.07.108
10. Upadhyay UD, Raymond EG, Koenig LR, et al. Outcomes and safety of history-based screening for medication abortion: a retrospective multicenter cohort study. *JAMA Intern Med*. 2022; 182(5):482–491. https://doi.org/10.1001/jamainternmed.2022.0217
11. Allsworth JE. Telemedicine, medication abortion, and access after *Roe v. Wade*. *Am J Public Health*. 2022;112(8):1086–1088. https://doi.org/10.2105/AJPH.2022.306948
12. Baker CN. History and politics of medication abortion in the United States and the rise of telemedicine and self-managed abortion. *J Health Polit Policy Law*. 2023;48(4):485–510. https://doi.org/10.1215/03616878-10449941
13. Koenig LR, Ko J, Upadhyay UD. Virtual clinic telehealth abortion services in the United States one year after Dobbs: a landscape review [preprint]. Published online July 13, 2023. https://doi.org/10.2196/preprints.50749
14. Raymond EG, Grossman D, Mark A, et al. Commentary: no-test medication abortion: a sample protocol for increasing access during a pandemic and beyond. *Contraception*. 2020;101(6):361–366. https://doi.org/10.1016/j.contraception.2020.04.005
15. American College of Obstetricians and Gynecologists' Committee on Practice Bulletins—Gynecology, Society of Family Planning. Medication abortion up to 70 days of gestation: ACOG Practice Bulletin, Number 225. *Obstet Gynecol*. 2020;136(4):e31–e47. https://doi.org/10.1097/AOG.0000000000004082
16. Godfrey EM, Thayer EK, Fiastro AE, Aiken ARA, Gomperts R. Family medicine provision of online medication abortion in three US states during COVID-19. *Contraception*. 2021;104(1):54–60. https://doi.org/10.1016/j.contraception.2021.04.026
17. Kaiser Family Foundation. The availability and use of medication abortion. September, 2023. Available at: https://www.kff.org/womens-health-policy/fact-sheet/the-availability-and-use-of-medication-abortion. Accessed December 13, 2023.
18. Kerestes C, Delafield R, Elia J, Chong E, Kaneshiro B, Soon R. "It was close enough, but it wasn't close enough": a qualitative exploration of the impact of direct-to-patient telemedicine abortion on access to abortion care. *Contraception*. 2021;104(1):67–72. https://doi.org/10.1016/j.contraception.2021.04.028
19. Kerestes C, Delafield R, Elia J, Shochet T, Kaneshiro B, Soon R. Person-centered, high-quality care from a distance: a qualitative study of patient experiences of TelAbortion, a model for direct-to-patient medication abortion by mail in the United States. *Perspect Sex Reprod Health*. 2022;54(4):177–187. https://doi.org/10.1363/psrh.12210
20. Chong E, Shochet T, Raymond E, et al. Expansion of a direct-to-patient telemedicine abortion service in the United States and experience during the COVID-19 pandemic. *Contraception*. 2021; 104(1):43–48. https://doi.org/10.1016/j.contraception.2021.03.019
21. Koenig LR, Becker A, Ko J, Upadhyay UD. The role of telehealth in promoting equitable abortion access in the United States: spatial analysis. *JMIR Public Health and Surveillance*. 2023;9:e45671. https://doi.org/10.2196/45671
22. Fiastro AE, Sanan S, Jacob-Files E, et al. Remote delivery in reproductive health care: operation of direct-to-patient telehealth medication abortion services in diverse settings. *Ann Fam Med*. 2022; 20(4):336–342. https://doi.org/10.1370/afm.2821
23. Stephens J, Greenberg GM. Asynchronous telehealth. *Prim Care*. 2022;49(4):531–541. https://doi.org/10.1016/j.pop.2022.05.004
24. Jones RK, Jerman J. Characteristics and circumstances of US women who obtain very early and second-trimester abortions. *PLoS One*. 2017; 12(1):e0169969. https://doi.org/10.1371/journal.pone.0169969
25. Eberly LA, Kallan MJ, Julien HM, et al. Patient characteristics associated with telemedicine access for primary and specialty ambulatory care during the COVID-19 pandemic. *JAMA Netw Open*. 2020;3(12):e2031640. https://doi.org/10.1001/jamanetworkopen.2020.31640
26. Aiken A, Lohr PA, Lord J, Ghosh N, Starling J. Effectiveness, safety and acceptability of no-test medical abortion (termination of pregnancy) provided via telemedicine: a national cohort study. *BJOG*. 2021;128(9):1464–1474. https://doi.org/10.1111/1471-0528.16668

Unpacked Cochrane Review on Masks: A Further Look

Jesper M. Kivelä, DMedSc

ABOUT THE AUTHOR

Jesper M. Kivelä is with the HUS Diagnostic Center, Helsinki University Hospital and University of Helsinki, Finland.

Gurbaxani et al. tried to unpack an updated Cochrane review on physical interventions to reduce respiratory infections.[1] Only a minority of 78 trials included in the Cochrane review covered masks; thus, one should apply some care when considering the review's overall conclusions.[2] Also, the review included many cluster-randomized trials on masks—thus, touching the source control aspect, which is contrary to what Gurbaxani et al. indicated when they cited the article in *The Conversation* (https://bit.ly/47TjPQI).

Although the Cochrane review authors judged that only two of 78 trials had low risk of bias in all domains, risk of bias was low for sequence generation in seven or low for allocation concealment in four trials in mask versus no mask comparison for influenza or COVID-19–like illness (nine trials).[2] A random-effects metaregression based on these nine trials using sequence generation or allocation concealment (high or unclear vs low risk of bias) as a covariate yields ratio of risk ratios of 0.84 (95% confidence interval [CI] = 0.53, 1.32) and 0.88 (95% CI = 0.66, 1.18), respectively. A systematic review of meta-epidemiological studies has indicated that compared to trials with clear and adequate sequence generation and allocation concealment, randomized trials with unclear or inadequate sequence generation or allocation concealment tend to overestimate effect size, especially with subjective outcomes.[3]

Two randomized trials on severe acute respiratory syndrome coronavirus 2 (SARS-CoV-2) were included in the updated Cochrane review that compared masks to no masks (a third trial conducted in Guinea-Bissau was listed as ongoing).[4,5] The larger trial conducted in Bangladesh was judged by the Cochrane review authors to have more risk of bias domains than the smaller trial conducted in Denmark (namely, DANMASK-19), which is similar to another quality assessment (i.e., fair vs good quality).[6]

Two additional analyses based on DANMASK-19 were overlooked by Gurbaxani et al.: a per-protocol analysis that excluded participants who reported noncompliance (odds ratio [OR] = 0.84; 95% CI = 0.55, 1.26) and a post hoc analysis that included participants who reported wearing masks exactly as instructed (OR = 0.93; 95% CI = 0.56, 1.54).[5] As evident, both results are in line with the main result (OR = 0.82; 95% CI = 0.54, 1.23).

Nonetheless, a Bayesian random-effects meta-analysis of these two randomized trials resulted in a risk ratio of 0.91 (95% credible interval = 0.63, 1.33) with a probability of 73% for some benefit with masks to reduce SARS-CoV-2 infections.[7]

Public health should be informed by systematic and impartial evaluation of the best available evidence on masks despite what the results show. AJPH

Letters to the editor referring to a recent *AJPH* article are encouraged up to 3 months after the article's appearance. By submitting a letter to the editor, the author gives permission for its publication in *AJPH*. Letters should not duplicate material being published or submitted elsewhere. The editors reserve the right to edit and abridge letters and to publish responses. Text is limited to 400 words and 7 references. Submit online at www.editorialmanager.com/ajph. Queries should be addressed to the Editor-in-Chief, Alfredo Morabia, MD, PhD, at editorajph@apha.org.

CORRESPONDENCE

Correspondence should be sent to Jesper Kivelä, HUS Diagnostic Center, HUSLAB Building, Topeliuksenkatu 32, PO Box 720, 00290 Helsinki, Finland (e-mail: jesper.m.kivela@helsinki.fi). Reprints can be ordered at https://ajph.org by clicking the "Reprints" link.

PUBLICATION INFORMATION

Full Citation: Kivelä JM. Unpacked Cochrane review on masks: a further look. *Am J Public Health*. 2024;114(2):251–252.

Acceptance Date: November 5, 2023.

DOI: https://doi.org/10.2105/AJPH.2023.307526

CONFLICTS OF INTEREST

The author has no conflicts of interest.

REFERENCES

1. Gurbaxani BM, Hill AN, Patel P. Unpacking Cochrane's update on masks and COVID-19. *Am J Public Health*. 2023;113(10):1074–1078. https://doi.org/10.2105/AJPH.2023.307377
2. Jefferson T, Dooley L, Ferroni E, et al. Physical interventions to interrupt or reduce the spread of respiratory viruses. *Cochrane Database Syst Rev*. 2023;1(1):CD006207. https://doi.org/10.1002/14651858.CD006207.pub6
3. Page MJ, Higgins JPT, Clayton G, Sterne JAC, Hróbjartsson A, Savović J. Empirical evidence of study design biases in randomized trials: systematic review of meta-epidemiological studies. *PLoS One*. 2016;11(7):e0159267. https://doi.org/10.1371/journal.pone.0159267
4. Abaluck J, Kwong LH, Styczynski A, et al. Impact of community masking on COVID-19: a cluster-randomized trial in Bangladesh. *Science*. 2022;375(6577):eabi9069. https://doi.org/10.1126/science.abi9069
5. Bundgaard H, Bundgaard JS, Raaschou-Pedersen DET, et al. Effectiveness of adding a mask recommendation to other public health measures to prevent SARS-CoV-2 infection in Danish mask wearers: a randomized controlled trial. *Ann Intern Med*. 2021;174(3):335–343. https://doi.org/10.7326/M20-6817
6. Chou R, Dana T. Major update: masks for prevention of SARS-CoV-2 in health care and community settings—final update of a living, rapid review. *Ann Intern Med*. 2023;176(6):827–835. https://doi.org/10.7326/M23-0570
7. Kivelä JM. Re: Public health measures for COVID-19. *BMJ*. 2021;375:n2729. https://www.bmj.com/content/375/bmj.n2729/rr-3. Accessed January 3, 2024.

Gurbaxani et al. Respond

Brian M. Gurbaxani, PhD, Andrew N. Hill, PhD, and Pragna Patel, MD, MPH

ABOUT THE AUTHORS

Brian M. Gurbaxani and Pragna Patel are with the National Center for Immunization and Respiratory Diseases, Centers for Disease Control and Prevention (CDC), Atlanta, GA. B. M. Gurbaxani is also with the Departments of Electrical and Computer Engineering and Industrial and Systems Engineering, Georgia Institute of Technology, Atlanta. Andrew N. Hill is with the National Center for Emerging and Zoonotic Infectious Diseases, Division of Parasitic Diseases and Malaria, CDC, and the Department of Biostatistics and Bioinformatics, Rollins School of Public Health, Emory University, Atlanta. P. Patel is also with the Department of Medicine, Emory University.

We thank Jesper M. Kivelä for his thoughtful response to our article[1]; we agree that "methods matter"[2] and warrant careful consideration. We did not unpack all of Cochrane's update on masks,[3] but focused on the studies applicable to severe acute respiratory syndrome coronavirus 2 (SARS-CoV-2).[1]

Kivelä demonstrates that inclusion of studies deemed to have higher risk of bias in terms of sequence generation or allocation concealment (which prevent selection bias) distorts the relative risk of viral respiratory illness away from the null, but his accompanying confidence intervals indicate statistical nonsignificance. Therefore, his point is unclear. For the two largest studies (each at least an order of magnitude larger than the other seven that Kivelä reanalyzes), the effect sizes for masks either were very small and corroborated by our modeling results in the Abaluck et al.[4] study, as we discussed,[1] or were expected to be small given the comparatively much lower mask use (24%) in the treatment arm of the Alfelali et al.[5] study. Thus, the absence of a statistically significant result was not unexpected given the barely observable effect in the largest studies.

This reiterates the main conclusion of our original study[6] and the comment on the Cochrane review[1]—that is, that modeling is crucial to interpreting randomized controlled trial results for masks. Moreover, Cochrane's meta-analyses use fixed and random effects methods of evaluation; these are inappropriate tools for masks because masks do not have a fixed effect size. The effectiveness of masks depends on many variables, such as the prevalence and basic reproductive number (R_0) of the virus, the level of usage and type and fit of masks, and the dynamics of the epidemic. More pertinently, nonpharmaceutical interventions are instituted at a population level to flatten the epidemic curve and reduce the herd immunity threshold. If the R_0 of the virus is high, the reduction in total infections attributable to masks over the course of the randomized controlled trial could be quite small, but the lengthening of time to infection would not be.

The impact of masks, or other nonpharmaceutical interventions, on epidemic dynamics is important, but cannot be adequately evaluated in a meta-analysis. A time-to-infection analysis would likely produce a more robust evaluation of the effect of masks. Masks have a clear, causal mechanism of operation: their effect is certainly not zero[1] but is also dynamic and not fixed. Models show that masks can have a substantial population impact and can inform both individual wearers and recommendations for mask use by public health officials. AJPH

CORRESPONDENCE

Correspondence should be sent to Brian M. Gurbaxani, Centers for Disease Control and Prevention, 1600 Clifton Rd NE, Bldg 24, 7th Floor, MS H24-7, Atlanta, GA 30333 (e-mail: buw8@cdc.gov). Reprints can be ordered at http://www.ajph.org by clicking the "Reprints" link.

PUBLICATION INFORMATION

Full Citation: Gurbaxani BM, Hill AN, Patel P. Gurbaxani et al. respond. *Am J Public Health*. 2024;114(2):252–253.

Acceptance Date: November 5, 2023.

DOI: https://doi.org/10.2105/AJPH.2023.307527

CONTRIBUTORS

B. M. Gurbaxani conceptualized and wrote the initial draft of the letter and formulated the statistical response. A. N. Hill verified J. M. Kivelä's statistical computations and formulated our response to them, and contributed to the overall statistical response. A. N. Hill and P. Patel contributed to the writing. P. Patel added an epidemiological perspective. All authors reviewed and approved the final version.

ACKNOWLEDGMENTS

The authors would like to thank Noelle-Angelique M. Molinari, PhD, the associate director for Epidemiologic Science, Coronavirus and Other Respiratory Viruses Division, for her support of this letter.

Note. The findings and conclusions in this article are those of the authors and do not necessarily represent the official position of the CDC.

CONFLICTS OF INTEREST

The authors have no conflicts of interest to declare.

REFERENCES

1. Gurbaxani BM, Hill AN, Patel P. Unpacking Cochrane's update on masks and COVID-19. *Am J Public Health*. 2023;113(10):1074–1078. https://doi.org/10.2105/AJPH.2023.307377
2. Kivelä JM. Do methods in meta-analyses matter? *Eur J Pediatr*. 2022;181(11):3989. https://doi.org/10.1007/s00431-022-04618-1
3. Jefferson T, Dooley L, Ferroni E, et al. Physical interventions to interrupt or reduce the spread of respiratory viruses. *Cochrane Database Syst Rev*. 2023;1(1):CD006207. https://doi.org/10.1002/14651858.CD006207.pub6
4. Abaluck J, Kwong LH, Styczynski A, et al. Impact of community masking on COVID-19: a cluster-randomized trial in Bangladesh. *Science*. 2022;375(6577):eabi9069. https://doi.org/10.1126/science.abi9069
5. Alfelali M, Haworth EA, Barasheed O, et al. Facemask against viral respiratory infections among Hajj pilgrims: a challenging cluster-randomized trial. *PLoS One*. 2020;15(10):e0240287. https://doi.org/10.1371/journal.pone.0240287
6. Gurbaxani BM, Hill AN, Paul P, Prasad PV, Slayton RB. Evaluation of different types of face masks to limit the spread of SARS-CoV-2: a modeling study. *Sci Rep*. 2022;12(1):8630. https://doi.org/10.1038/s41598-022-11934-x